HERBS
that
WORK

HERBS

that

WORK

The Scientific Evidence
of Their Healing Powers

DAVID ARMSTRONG

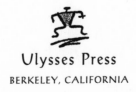

Ulysses Press
BERKELEY, CALIFORNIA

Published by: Ulysses Press
                P.O. Box 3440
                Berkeley, CA 94703
                www.ulyssespress.com

Library of Congress Catalog Card Number: 99-69194
ISBN: 1-56975-211-7

Printed in Canada by Transcontinental Printing

10 9 8 7 6 5 4 3 2 1

Editor: Mark Woodworth
Cover Design: Sarah Levin, Leslie Henriques
Herb illustration on page 12 is by QuickArt®, copyright by Wheeler Arts
Editorial and production staff: Marin Van Young, David Wells, Lily Chou
Indexer: Sayre Van Young

Distributed in the United States by Publishers Group West,
in Canada by Raincoast Books, and in Great Britain and Europe
by Airlift Book Company.

TABLE OF CONTENTS

Introduction   ix

PART 1: The Herbs that Work   1

PART 2: The Dubious Dozen   167

Appendix   183
Glossary   189
Weights and Measures Chart   193
Metric Conversion Chart   193
Bibliography   194
Index   196
About the Author   208

Note from the Publisher

This book has been written and published strictly for informational purposes, and in no way should it be used as a substitute for consultation with your medical doctor or health care professional. All facts in this book came from medical files, clinical journals, scientific publications, personal interviews, published trade books, self-published materials by experts, magazine articles, and the personal-practice experiences of the authorities quoted or sources cited. You should not consider educational material herein to be the practice of medicine or to replace consultation with a physician or other medical practitioner. The author and publisher are providing you with information in this work so that you can have the knowledge and can choose, at your own risk, to act on that knowledge. The author and publisher also urge all readers to be aware of their health status and to consult health professionals before beginning any health program, including changes in dietary habits. **Be sure to tell your doctor and pharmacist about *all* medications you take, both prescription drugs and over-the-counter products. Some herbs (even some teas) and supplements may interact with prescribed medications.**

INTRODUCTION

All of a sudden, herbs seem to be everywhere. They crowd the shelves of drugstores and health food stores in capsules, tea bags, and tinctures. They are prominent ingredients in supermarket weight-loss formulas and skin-care products. They dominate aisle after aisle of nutritional centers in shopping malls. They're even sprinkled into potato chips, cereals, and fruit drinks. Indeed, looking at the commercial and medicinal landscape of the United States at the dawn of the 21st century, one could hardly be blamed for concluding that echinacea, saw palmetto, and St. John's wort are as all-American as Prozac, burgers, and fries.

In fact, the sale and use of herbal products has been growing in the U.S. since the 1970s, when a renaissance began of holistic medicine, skepticism toward Big Science, and the understandable desire for kinder, gentler means of treating disease and discomfort. In the late 1990s, the renaissance reached critical mass. In 1998, according to the *New York Times*, Americans spent $27.2 billion on alternative health care—vitamin and mineral supplements, acupuncture, chiropractic, and others—nearly twice as much as in 1994.

But while the growth in sales has been healthy, there's an unhealthy lack of reliable information, at least in the U.S., about just what all that money's buying. There are several reasons for this, and they reinforce one another:

First, U.S. medical doctors, infatuated with antibiotics and other postwar laboratory "miracle" drugs, practically stopped studying phytomedicines, that is, medicines derived from plants, let alone recommending them to patients. Moreover, the U.S. Food and Drug Administration, the major regulatory agency, presently classifies herbal drugs not as medicines but dietary supplements; the FDA—at the behest of Congress through the Dietary Supplement Health and Education Act of 1994—doesn't require proof that plant drugs actually work, nor does it require that herbal remedies undergo the same rigorous premarket testing that standard pharmaceutical drugs must pass before they can be sold. Finally, American pharmaceutical firms don't voluntarily test herbal medicines on their own, because they're unable to patent the plants found in nature; that means the $350 million to $500 million that companies spend to bring each and every new drug to market is too much to spend on nonproprietary herbs. Without a patent, pharmaceutical firms fear they won't recoup their huge investment in drug research and development. Thus, for a variety of reasons, doctors, government regulators, and drug companies all fall down on their responsibilities to provide American consumers with reliable, continually updated information about herbal medicine.

All this puts crucial responsibility on consumers to educate themselves about what herbal medicines are, how they work, what their potential benefits and risks are, and even how to buy them. That would seem to be easy enough, in the information age. But, face it, anyone can throw up a website about herbs or anything else, and say practically anything, with or without documentation. Media accounts of herbs are often oversimplified, resulting in reports of medical breakthroughs that aren't, or scare stories that wildly exaggerate the dangers of herbs (although risks do exist, especially for the uninformed). There's no shortage of books about herbs, but many herbals, as such books are called, fall into one of two categories: the boosterism of the true believer, and the cynicism of the self-dramatizing "quackbuster." Neither approach is useful.

This book seeks to avoid both extremes, and to meld the American experience with the best practices of herbal healers abroad. Indeed, to find the most advanced scientific updates on herbs as medicines, one must look beyond the U.S. border, which is what I've done in preparing this book.

The best place to look is Germany. German medical schools incorporate the study of herbs in their core curriculum, and 70 percent of German M.D.s prescribe herbal drugs in addition to conventional drugs. Herbal medicine in Germany is mainstream, not fringe. As a consequence, German healers and consumers have long-standing and wide-ranging experience with herbs, which are sold medicinally in three forms: as prescription drugs, as over-the-counter drugs, and as nonprescription drugs available only from licensed pharmacists.

Even with their extensive experience, German authorities decided they needed to know more about herbal drugs. In 1978, the federal government of what was then West Germany decided to weed out the worst of the country's plant-derived medicines. The government appointed a blue-ribbon panel of experts to evaluate herbal remedies and decide which ones work and which ones don't. The panel, called Commission E, had 24 members and consisted of medical doctors, pharmacists, toxicologists, pharmacologists, and laypeople. It issued scientific monographs—profiles—of nearly 400 herbs as well as fixed-combination drugs made from two or more herbs. Commission E issued monographs from 1983 to 1995. The Commission approved 254 herbs, and it nixed medicinal use of 126 herbs. It also approved 66 fixed-combination herbal formulas and turned thumbs down on 6 others. (Most fixed-combination German herbal drugs aren't sold in the U.S.).

No human endeavor is all-seeing and all-inclusive, but Germany's Commission E is widely acknowledged by herbal authorities in the Western world as the scientific benchmark for phyto-

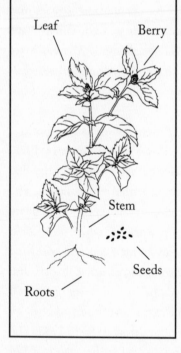

Herb (pronounced urb*):
Any part of any plant for
which humans find a
personal use.*

Leaf

Berry

Stem

Seeds

Roots

medicines: drugs derived from plants. Varro E. Tyler, Ph.D., the gray eminence of herbal medicine in the U.S., writes that the report is "the most accurate information available in the entire world on the safety and efficacy of herbs and phytomedicines." American herbal author Steven B. Karch, M.D., agrees, commenting that "the findings of Commission E represent the single most reliable source for such information."

This book is grounded in Commission E's findings, providing profiles of the 75 most popular and potentially useful herbs approved by the commission and offering critical looks at 12 common herbs it didn't approve. But while I start with Commission E's evaluations, I don't end with them. This book enlarges the frame of reference for selected herbs, cross-referencing Commission E's findings with those of other herbal authorities. In the process, I add to Commission E's findings and, in a very few instances, where the weight of international scientific evidence seems to go against the commission, I depart from its conclusions.

I'm not the first to cite Commission E's report. In 1998, the American Botanical Council, an herb industry trade group based in Austin, Texas, published an English translation of the report. This exhaustive effort, a $189.00, 685-page hardcover volume targeted at health-care professionals, is a valuable addition to the reference shelves of medical libraries. Thoughtful American herbals published in 1998 and 1999 cited Commission E's report but did so mainly by way of referencing the commission as additional relevant information. This book reverses the usual approach, beginning with Commission E and building on its work. I summarize the commission's scientific findings for the nonspecialist in plain English, in an inexpensive, concise, portable form that virtually anyone will find easy to carry to the food market or the drugstore. Additionally, I provide expanded consumer information on eight selected herbs that I call the "Power 8."

It's important to point out that Commission E's monographs don't meet the USFDA's super-strict requirement of "absolute certainty" for drug safety and efficacy, based on double-blind clinical studies of human beings. In fact, Commission E draws on human studies when available, melding clinical trials with the long empirical use of herbs in Germany, giving weight to the testimony of physicians, druggists, and patients themselves. It also draws on unpublished proprietary studies of specific herbal medicines by the German pharmaceutical industry. At the end of the day, the commission embraces a "reasonable certainty" principle—not the USFDA's absolute certainty with regard to drugs that it approves for safety and efficacy.

Germany may not have developed a perfect system, but I think it has the best system of any advanced nation for using and evaluating herbal medicines. Herbal medicines are, of course, used around the world and have been since the beginning of time. They were staples of Native American societies over centuries, are very popular among India's Ayurvedic healers, and are widely used in East Asia. I myself, for example, have visited a sprawling herb market in Xian, China, where whole, raw herbs were stacked for sale under weepy skies in the open air, and lunched at a sleek restaurant in Singapore, called the Imperial Herbal Restaurant, where medicinal herbs were added to every dish. My favorite was the stewed duck with peas and hawthorn, an herb covered in this book; hawthorn is added, according to the restaurant menu, to help with "digesting fat, promoting energy flow, and dispensing coagulations." However, many herbal medicines in Asia contain up to a dozen ingredients, and some include minerals and animal body parts; the Singapore restaurant, for example, also displayed the ready-to-eat, dried bodies of scorpions in wicked-looking, black heaps. Such drugs are not the relatively simple and straightforward medicines favored in Germany; nor have most been systematically evaluated, like German drugs. Germany and Commission E have raised the bar for the modern use of herbal medicine.

FYI: You should know that I'm a journalist and author, not a physician. I have no ties, financial or otherwise, to the herb trade or pharmaceutical industry. I believe that the decision to use herbs medicinally or not to use them is strictly up to you. If after perusing this book you decide to try medicinal herbs, use your common sense: Read product labels carefully. Look for the presence of standardized amounts of active ingredients on labels, as well as the manufacturer's toll-free telephone number, website, or mailing address, should you need more information. Question salesclerks, but don't accept their answers on faith; most are well-meaning, and some are experienced with herbs, but many are poorly trained. Lastly, keep it simple: If you buy anything, go for single-herb preparations, not complicated, aggressively marketed, "synergistic" combinations.

Part 1

The Herbs that Work

ALOE

Aloe barbadensis

Aloe is a succulent shrub and member of the lily family. Native to southern Africa, and commonly known as aloe vera, it's often used in gel form to heal burns. In German medicine, aloe is taken internally and is valued as a laxative. One way or another, it has been used medicinally for a long time. The ancient Greeks used aloe; in fact, it was prized by Alexander the Great, who used aloe to treat the burns and wounds of soldiers in his conquering armies.

Potential Health Benefits

Commission E approved aloe for just one use: as a laxative. Indeed, *aloe barbadensis* is a straightforward, naturally based alternative to synthetically made laxatives with long lists of ingredients. The medically useful part of the plant is the juice from aloe's fleshy leaves, which stimulates the colon. Besides being used to soothe sunburn and regular burns, aloe vera gel is a popular ingredient in cosmetics.

Scientific Evidence

Commission E published monographs on this herb in 1985 and 1993. In both cases, commission studies found that aloe is reliable and effective; scientists attribute pharmacological action of the herb to its 1,8-dihydroxy-anthracene derivatives. Other health writers cite exciting possible uses for aloe. In the *National Geographic* book *Nature's Medicine*, Joel L. Swerdlow, Ph.D., writes: "In laboratory tests, aloe-emodin (an ingredient in aloe) has shown signs of being able to combat leukemia." Aloe juice has also been tested as a treatment for diabetes, with mixed results. A 1997 study published in the journal *Phytomedicine* found that 77 people who took 1 tablespoon of aloe juice twice daily for up to 42 days had a significant reduction in blood sugar levels. Another study, published in *Psychotherapy Research* in 1994, found no helpful action against diabetes. In any case, aloe's laxative powers are long-established; if anything, North American herbalists consider it stronger than it has to be, often recommending gentler laxatives.

How to Use the Herb

For internal use, aloe is taken as a powder made from the dried latex of its leaves and usually mixed with water or an alcohol-based extract and swallowed. The daily dose is 20-30 milligrams, divided into 2 or 3 separate doses.

Consumer Products Available

Aloe is available in health food stores as an extract or powder, and in health food stores and drugstores as aloe vera gel. The product label should specify "stabilized" gel for best results on the skin. Aloe juice is sometimes marketed as a virtual panacea and even as a cure for AIDS. Commission E and reputable herbalists stop well short of making such claims, which the American health writer Andrew Weil, M.D., calls "sheer fantasy."

Potential Dangers

Long-term internal use of aloe juice, more than the recommended one to two weeks, could cause an electrolyte imbalance or a potassium deficiency. Aloe shouldn't be given to children under 12 or used by nursing mothers or during pregnancy. Overdoses can cause intestinal cramps. Commission E concluded that "The preparation should be used only if no effect can be obtained through change of diet or use of bulk-forming products." There's no risk to using aloe externally on the skin.

ANISE SEED

Pimpinella anisum

This pleasant-tasting plant, native to Egypt, is now cultivated in many parts of the world. It's related to carrots and parsley, but tastes so much like licorice that it's used to flavor licorice candy and liqueur. The medicinal part of anise is the dried fruit, commonly referred to as seeds.

Potential Health Benefits

Commission E endorsed preparations made from anise seeds to treat upset stomach and clear the lungs of phlegm. The commission found that anise also has antibiotic qualities. Anise is used to treat bronchitis, fever, and sore throat.

Scientific Evidence

The essential oil made from anise seeds includes the chemical anethole and chemicals creosol and alpha-pinene, which make anise effective as an expectorant. American health writer Steven B. Karch, M.D., writes: "Clinical studies of anise are very few in number, but results of laboratory studies suggest that anise is an anti-inflammatory agent and a very good anti-oxidant. Extracts of anise inhibit the growth of certain tumors, particularly colon cancer." More study of this potentially important use is undoubtedly needed.

How to Use the Herb

Commission E recommends an average daily dose of 3 grams of the drug or 0.3 grams of the essential oil, both taken orally. Anise tea can be made by crushing 1 teaspoonful of anise seeds and steeping 10–20 minutes in hot water; take the tea 3 times per day. American health writer Michael Castleman additionally recommends ½–1 teaspoonful of tincture, taken up to 3 times per day as a treatment for cough, bronchitis and asthma, and as a digestive aid.

Consumer Products Available

Anise seeds are available in health food stores, as are tinctures.

Potential Dangers

Allergy to the anethole in anise can irritate the skin and stomach. No overdose levels are listed, and there are no known interactions with other drugs, but note that anise seeds are contraindicated for children.

BELLADONNA

Atropa belladonna

Belladonna, from the Italian, meaning "beautiful lady," is a perennial herb containing the alkaloid atropine. The plant puts out purplish, bell-shaped flowers and black berries. Its popular name, deadly nightshade, signals that belladonna can indeed be a poison when used carelessly. Used correctly, it's an effective treatment for a range of maladies.

Potential Health Benefits

Extracts of the root and leaf are used to treat "spasms and colic-like pain in the gastrointestinal tract and bile ducts," according to Commission E. Belladonna extracts are also employed to dilate the pupil of the eye for eye examinations and eye surgery.

Scientific Evidence

Belladonna affects the brain and central nervous system, disrupting the effects of acetylocholine, a chemical messenger in the nervous system. Pharmacologists have found sedative effects and narcotic qualities in belladonna; it's also antispasmodic. Belladonna is effective as a local anesthetic. Homeopaths have used minute doses of belladonna to treat scarlet fever and thyroid disorders. Additionally, belladonna is an ingredient in prescription drugs such as Donnatal and Laugin.

How to Use the Herb

Carefully, under the supervision of a homeopathic doctor or herbalist.

As a leaf powder, the average single dose is 0.05–0.1 gram. Maximum single dose is 0.2 gram, equivalent to 0.6 milligram total alkaloids, calculated as hyoscyamine. Maximum daily dose is 0.6 gram, equivalent to 1.8 milligrams total alkaloids, calculated as hyoscyamine.

For belladonna root, the average single dose is 0.05 gram. The maximum single dose is 0.1 gram, equivalent to 0.5 milligrams total alkaloids, calculated as hyoscyamine. Maximum daily dose is 0.3 grams, equivalent to 1.5 total alkaloids, calculated as hyoscyamine.

For belladonna extract, the average single dose is 0.01 gram. Maximum single dose is 0.05 gram, equivalent to 0.73 milligrams total alkaloids, calculated as hyoscyamine. Maximum daily dose is 0.15 gram, equivalent to 2.2 milligrams total alkaloids, calculated as hyoscyamine.

Consumer Products Available

Powders and extracts are available in drugstores, and as ingredients in prescription drugs.

Potential Dangers

There are many, chiefly due to overdose: rapid heartbeat, difficulty urinating, restlessness, hallucinations, red and dry skin, prolonged dilation of the pupils, dry mouth. Belladonna can magnify the effects of prescription drugs such as Amantadine and Quinidine, and antidepressants Elavil, Pamelor, and Tofranil. Belladonna shouldn't be used by persons with narrow-angle glaucoma. It is also contraindicated for men with prostate problems.

BILBERRY FRUIT

Vaccinium myrtillus

Bilberry is a dwarf shrub of the heath family, named after the Danish word for "dark fruit." A native European plant, it's related to North American blueberries and cranberries. The bilberry shrub produces small, egg-shaped leaves, rose-colored flowers, and dark-blue berries. The berries (that is, the fruit) are the medicinal part of the plant, which is also called huckleberry or whortleberry.

Potential Health Benefits

Commission E endorses the dried, ripe fruit and preparations made from it for use against acute diarrhea and to soothe sore throats. Broad claims by some writers that bilberry prevents macular degeneration in the eye, promotes night vision, and serves as a super-saver of eyesight weren't addressed by Commission E.

Scientific Evidence

Bilberry preparations contain tannins, flavonoid glycosides, and anthocyanosides. Flavonoids and anthocyanosides are credited with producing the salutary health benefits of red wine and grape juice. In laboratory tests, flavonoids prevent the oxidization of low-density cholesterol, which suggests they might be useful for preventing coronary heart disease. Without citing specifics, health writer James A. Duke, Ph.D., alludes to research in the 1990s that he says "has demonstrated bilberry's efficacy in treating circulatory complications due to diabetes or hypertension, bruising, capillary fragility, varicose veins, hemorrhoids, and Raynaud's disease." Commission E's report, published in 1994, doesn't address these much broader uses of bilberry fruit. Bilberry leaf was listed as unapproved by the commission, which favors the fruit.)

How to Use the Herb

For internal use, take a daily dose of 20–60 grams, or 1 to 2 ounces of the dried berry. Bilberry tea can be made by putting 1–2 teaspoonfuls of crushed berries in cold water, soaking for 10 minutes, and straining. Supplements set at 80–100 milligrams, taken 3 times per day, are recommended by a variety of health writers. James A. Duke recommends capsules that are standardized to 25 percent anthocyanosides.

Consumer Products Available

Bilberry is available in health food stores and drugstores, as capsules, drops, extracts, and mashed, dried berries.

Potential Dangers

Commission E assessed only bilberry fruit, finding no contraindications, interactions with other drugs, or side effects. If diarrhea persists for 3–4 days, consult a physician. Bilberry leaf, not approved by the commission, is considered potentially toxic by some herbalists.

BITTER ORANGE PEEL

Citrus aaurantium

The bitter orange, native to Asia but now widely grown, is the small, unripened fruit of a tropical evesgreen. Used to flavor teas and liqueurs, the fresh and dried peel of the fruit is also medicinally useful.

Potential Health Benefits

Bitter orange peel and its preparations can restore lost appetite and quiet an upset stomach.

Scientific Evidence

The peel contains essential oil and bitter principles.

How to Use the Herb

The crushed peel can be taken in tea, used until symptoms have eased or disappeared, which is the case with other modes of administration, too. The daily dosage recommended by Commission E is 4–6 grams of the dried peel, 2–3 grams of tincture, or 1–2 grams of extract.

Consumer Products Available

Teas, tinctures, and extracts are sold in health food stores.

Potential Dangers

Light-skinned individuals may find themselves more sensitive to sunlight. The peel can irritate the skin when handled.

BLACK COHOSH ROOT

Cimicifuga racemosa

A perennial herb used in traditional Native American medicine, black cohosh is also called squaw root and snake root. Indian healers used it to treat rattlesnake bite. It was a prime ingredient in the 19th-century version of the patent medicine Lydia Pinkham's Vegetable Compound, which was concocted for "female disorders," and still is—although black cohosh isn't listed on the label of the surviving version of Lydia Pinkham's. In Chinese medicine, black cohosh is called sheng ma.

Potential Health Benefits

Commission E approves black cohosh root as a treatment for menstrual discomfort and premenstrual syndrome and as a means of easing the mood swings and hot flashes of menopause. The commission didn't evaluate its usefulness for snakebite or endorse the herb for neurological conditions.

Scientific Evidence

Black cohosh works by suppressing luteinizing hormone and serving as an estrogen replacement. In one study of 60 women under 40 years of age who had had hysterectomies, black cohosh extract proved as effective as standard pharmaceutical drugs in easing menopause-like symptoms, although Commission E does not recommend using the herb for longer than six months. The only catch was, black cohosh took longer to produce an effect. Research published in 1991 in the journal *Planta Medica* and a 1997 study in the *Journal of Women's Health* reported that the herb has proven effective in treating symptoms of menopause. Health writers caution that since black cohosh doesn't contain estrogen, it has no power to prevent osteoporosis or heart disease. Still, results so far have been encouraging enough to prompt American herbal writer Varro E. Tyler, Ph.D., to write: "Further studies on this useful herb are warranted."

How to Use the Herb

Daily doses of extract, which are taken orally, are set at 40 milligrams by Commission E. Other sources also recommend up to 1 teaspoonful of tincture per day.

Consumer Products Available

Black cohosh is available in tinctures, tablets, and extracts in health food stores, drugstores, and supermarkets.

Potential Dangers

Commission E cites gastric distress as a side effect, but found no interactions with other drugs. Other sources say the herb can cause headaches and slow the heartbeat. Commission E concludes that pregnant women should not use black cohosh and advises others not to use black cohosh for more than six months.

BLACKBERRY LEAF

Rubus fruitcosuss

The humble blackberry—thorny, fruit-bearing, the creeping bramble found in gardens and backyards and in the wild—has little-appreciated medical applications. The medicinally available properties are in the leaf of this common plant, which is a relative of the rose and the raspberry.

Potential Health Benefits

The dried leaf is used to treat acute diarrhea and for soothing sore throat.

Scientific Evidence

The tannins in blackberry leaves have a drying, astringent quality useful for treating diarrhea. Blackberry isn't the subject of extensive scientific testing. Commission E's recommendations are drawn from the long empirical use of blackberry in German medicine.

How to Use the Herb

To make a tea, pour boiling water over 2 teaspoonfuls and steep for 10 minutes; the tea can also double as mouthwash. Commission E recommends ingestion of 4–5 grams of dried leaf per day for medical use. Health writer Michael Castleman recommends up to 2 teaspoonfuls of tincture per day to treat diarrhea or soothe a sore throat.

Consumer Products Available

Tea bags and dried leaves are available in health food stores.

Potential Dangers

Blackberry leaf is safe. There are no known contraindications, interactions with drugs, or side effects. Sensitive individuals can experience gastric distress because of the tannins in blackberry, although leaves have lower concentrations of tannins than does the root.

BREWER'S YEAST
Saccharomyces cerevisiae

All right, it tastes dreadful, but it's useful. The humble yeast is a single-cell organism—a fungus—that grows on starchy, sugary substances such as the grains used in baking and in brewing beer. Commission E studied brewer's yeast, a by-product of beer-making.

Potential Health Benefits

Commission E endorsed brewer's yeast to treat diarrhea, to fight chronic acne, and to restore lost appetite. North American researchers say the chromium in brewer's yeast helps ease symptoms of diabetes and raise levels of "good" HDL cholesterol, but Commission E didn't cite such far-ranging uses. Additionally, brewer's yeast is high in protein, which accounts for half its weight, so it's a good nutritional supplement for some people. Its high vitamin B_{12} content makes brewer's yeast a useful supplement for vegetarians.

Scientific Evidence

Abundant B vitamins and a broad range of minerals make brewer's yeast a useful ingredient in a prevention-minded diet or as a therapeutic agent. Brewer's yeast knocks out the nasty *E. coli* bacteria that cause diarrhea. Commission E reports that brewer's yeast reduced toxins from *vibrio cholerae* by 40 percent. "In animal studies," the commission reports, "the secretory immunoglobulin was increased in the gastrointestinal tract after oral intake of brewer's yeast." That's a good thing—it helps restore the appetite.

How to Use the Herb

Stir flakes or powdered yeast into water or juice, or sprinkle it on soups, salads, cereal, and popcorn. For treating diarrhea, Commission E recommends taking 250–500 milligrams per day. If you're going on a trip and want to prevent traveler's diarrhea, start taking brewer's yeast five days before departure. The daily dose for chronic acne is 750 milligrams.

Consumer Products Available

Health food stores and supermarkets sell powdered brewer's yeast, flakes, and tablets with standardized doses.

Potential Dangers

If diarrhea persists for more than two days, or if there's blood in the stool, get medical attention. Yeast shouldn't be given to infants. If flatulence or other gastric distress develops, you're taking too much; reduce the dose or increase the amount of liquid you're washing it down with. The American Botanical Council cautions that "simultaneous intake of MAO inhibitors may cause increased blood pressure."

CAMPHOR

Cinnamomum camphora

The camphor tree is a large evergreen native to Japan and Taiwan. It's the source of a volatile crystalline substance, also called camphor, which is distilled from the wood of the tree. Camphor gives mainstream preparations such as Vicks VapoRub their characteristic strong smell.

Potential Health Benefits

Used internally, camphor clears mucous from the upper respiratory tract. Inhaled in a steam preparation, it opens clogged nasal passages and eases bronchial coughs. Rubbed on the skin, it stimulates local circulation.

Scientific Evidence

Commission E offers little hard information on how camphor works, but it gives an unambiguous endorsement for both internal and external use to ease the symptoms of colds and flu, based on good results from long-time use of the herb in German medicine.

How to Use the Herb

Camphor is available in salves rubbed on the skin and liquid for inhaling or swallowing. For external use in stimulating circulation, the commission recommends 10–20 percent camphor in semisolid preparations and 1–10 percent camphor in spirits. For internal use against symptoms of colds and flu, the average daily dose can range from 30 to 300 milligrams.

Consumer Products Available

Camphor is available in salves and liquids in health food stores, drugstores, and supermarkets.

Potential Dangers

Don't use camphor for infants and small children. Sensitive adults can get contact eczema from this powerful substance. Overdoses can cause spasms and difficulty breathing.

CARAWAY SEED

Carum carvi

Caraway is well-known as a flavoring agent for rye bread, pastries, and liqueurs. It also has a health history going back some 5,000 years, and was cultivated in ancient Egypt. Both the aromatic seeds and the oil of caraway, a biennial plant native to Europe, are used medicinally. The oil is taken from the dried, ripe fruit of the plant (called the seeds).

Potential Health Benefits

Commission E endorses caraway oil and seed for treating upset stomach, bloating, and fullness. The commission also praised caraway for its antispasmotic qualities and ability to destroy microbes. Folklore credits caraway with the ability to improve lactation in nursing mothers, a use that the commission didn't address.

Scientific Evidence

The chemicals limonene and carvone are credited by researchers for caraway's ability to calm the smooth muscles of the digestive system. A 1996 double-blind, placebo-controlled study in Germany found that a mixture of caraway and peppermint oil was more effective at relieving indigestion than a placebo. On the whole, "Modern scientific studies are few and far between," writes American health writer Steven B. Karch, M.D., who adds "Anti-cancer effects have been demonstrated in laboratory animals, but not in humans."

How to Use the Herb

The daily dosage for caraway oil is 3–6 drops, in 2 divided doses. For seeds, a daily dose of 1.5–6.0 grams is recommended. Freshly crushed seeds can be used in infusions with 2–3 teaspoonfuls per cup of boiling water; steep for at least 10 minutes.

Consumer Products Available

Oil and seeds are available in health food stores, and seeds are sold in supermarkets.

Potential Dangers

There are no known contraindications, drug interactions, or major side effects, according to Commission E. *The PDR Family Guide to Natural Medicines & Healing Therapies* maintains that "large doses of caraway oil taken for established periods can cause liver or kidney damage."

CHAMOMILE FLOWER, GERMAN

Matricaria chamomilla

Chamomile is nothing if not versatile. The dried flowers of this plant, native to Europe and Asia, are used in teas, shampoos, and skin-care products. Most chamomile grown in North America is of the German variety, the same type studied by Commission E. There's also an English chamomile, also known as Roman chamomile, that the commission didn't approve for medicinal use. Chamomile is a relative of yarrow, another herb that won Commission E's seal of approval.

Potential Health Benefits

Commission E credits chamomile with calming gastrointestinal spasms and infections. Used externally, it combats bacterial skin conditions, deodorizes, and promotes the healing of wounds. Chamomile tea is a traditional favorite for bringing on sleep and tranquilizing jangled nerves.

Scientific Evidence

Chamomile flowers contain antispasmodics and anti-inflammatory agents. The active chemicals in chamomile are concentrated in the essential oil, which is an appealing blue color. Researchers credit a molecule called bioabolol with anti-inflammatory qualities and another molecule, apigenin, for chamomile's ability to settle the stomach. Apigenin is also credited by researchers with having a calming effect, accounting for chamomile's popularity in treating insomnia. Steven B. Karch, M.D., an American health author, writes: "A famous study published in the *Lancet* in 1993 found that high intakes of flavonoids, like the apigenin contained in chamomile, prevented heart disease. Even the vapors of chamomile oil appear to have beneficial effects. Studies in animals have shown that inhalation of chamomile vapor can, at least partly, block the hormonal response to stress."

How to Use the Herb

To make chamomile tea, pour boiling water over 1 tablespoon of dried flowers, steep for 5–10 minutes, and strain. Drink the tea 3 to 4 times per day between meals for upset stomach; the tea can also be used as a gargle for sore throats. For poultices and rinses, use a 3–10 percent infusion. For a fragrant bath, add 50 grams per 2½ gallons of water. Ointments and gels should contain 3–10 percent herb.

Consumer Products Available

Chamomile teas, flowers, and oil are available in health food stores and supermarkets.

Potential Dangers

Chamomile can trigger allergic reactions in persons sensitive to ragweed. But Commission E recorded no known contraindications, side effects, or drug interactions.

CHICORY

Cichorium intybus

Chicory, also known as succory, grows in Egypt, Asia, and the Americas, and is mentioned in ancient texts. Its blanched leaves are a popular addition to salads in our own day. Ground chicory also serves as a coffee substitute or is mixed with coffee to make a strong, pleasantly bitter brew. Healers use both the root and the above-ground parts of the plant.

Potential Health Benefits

Commission E finds chicory effective for stimulating appetite and alleviating dyspepsia (upset stomach).

Scientific Evidence

Chicory contains inulin, bitter principles, and pentosans and stimulates the liver to increase the production of bile, which in turn helps the body digest fat. As with other herbs that aren't studied extensively by scientists, Commission E draws its recommendations from empirical use. Additionally, a 1995 study published in the *Journal of Ethnopharmacology* found that a liquid extract of chicory root shows promise as a helpful antioxidant.

How to Use the Herb

For tea, use ½ teaspoon of the dried herb in boiling water, steep for 10 minutes, and strain. This is equivalent to 2 grams of the herb. Commission E says you may go as high as 3 grams per day overall.

Consumer Products Available

Chicory and coffee mixes, dried chicory leaves, and the whole plant are available in health food stores, herb shops, and supermarkets.

Potential Dangers

People with gallstones should always consult a physician before using chicory. In rare cases, touching the herb triggers allergic skin reactions.

CINNAMON BARK

Cinnamomum aromaticum

Cinnamon is almost as familiar as it's possible for an herb to be. It flavors toothpaste and mouthwash, is sprinkled on toast and into muffins, and is blended in teas. It's also used medicinally, especially the bark, and was known for its healing properties in ancient Egypt, China, and India. The bark is dried and turned into the sweet, yellow-brown spice used by millions of amateur and professional cooks and bakers.

Potential Health Benefits

Cinnamon bark calms unsettled stomachs, revives appetite, eases spasms of the gastrointestinal tract, and helps alleviate flatulence and that bloated feeling.

Scientific Evidence

Cinnamon oil found in bark stimulates the production of bile, helping the body break down fats. The chemical eugenol, found in the essential oil, is also present in cloves. Cinnamon has antibacterial qualities, which is why it's a fine ingredient in toothpaste, mouthwash, and gum. It also kills fungi. A German study found that cinnamon kills bacteria that cause urinary tract infections, while Japanese researchers concluded that it can help reduce high blood pressure—a point not often addressed in references to cinnamon.

How to Use the Herb

The daily dosage of bark recommended by the commission is 2–4 grams. The daily dose for essential oil is 0.05–0.2 grams of equivalent preparation. Cinnamon tea for upset stomachs is commonly taken 2 to 3 times per day with meals.

Consumer Products Available

Cinnamon sticks, capsules, teas, powders, and tinctures are sold in health food stores, herb shops, and supermarkets.

Potential Dangers

Pregnant women and people with ulcers shouldn't use cinnamon in medicinal amounts. The herb can cause skin allergies and irritate the inside of the mouth.

CLOVES
Syzygium aromaticum

As ancient as the tall tropical trees that produce them and as modern as the mouthwash Lavoris—which contains their oil—cloves are among the most popular herbs. Known for their instantly recognizable and powerful smell, cloves are the dried flower buds of the clove tree, grown commercially in Tanzania, Indonesia, and Sri Lanka. The essential oil is extracted from the flowers, leaves, and fruit.

Potential Health Benefits

Cloves' medicinal qualities are nearly as powerful as their smell. Undiluted oil of cloves is used as a local anesthetic in dentistry; at 1–5 percent essential oil, it's a cleansing mouthwash. Cloves also kill microbes in the mouth.

Scientific Evidence

The powdered and whole herb contain at least 14 percent essential oil. The oil is high in eugenol, which has antifungal and antiseptic qualities. Commission E additionally identifies antibacterial, antiviral, and antispasmotic properties in constituents of the oil. Studies of cloves published in such journals as *Planta Medica* in recent years underscore clove's ability to kill microbes and combat fungi and bacteria. In a report by U.S. scientists to the Food and Drug Administration, clove oil was singled out as the most effective active ingredient in commercial toothache remedies.

How to Use the Herb

For tea, take 1 teaspoon of powdered clove in a cup of boiling water, steep at least 10 minutes, and strain. A cotton swab dipped in clove oil will help relieve toothache temporarily.

Consumer Products Available

Powdered and whole cloves are sold in health food stores and supermarkets.

Potential Dangers

Clove oil in concentrated form can irritate sensitive mucosal tissue. Commission E found no drug interactions. Clove-spiked cigarettes, popular in Indonesia and specialty markets in other parts of the world, are just as carcinogenic as other kinds of smokes.

COLA NUT
Cola nitida

The nut of the cola plant—a tropical evergreen tree that can reach heights of 50 feet and more—is a familiar energizer in cola soft drinks. Actually, the nut gets its energy-generating powers from the same stimulant that launched thousands of coffee bars: caffeine.

Potential Health Benefits

Cola nut is used to banish mental and physical fatigue and increase concentration.

Scientific Evidence

The cola nut's caffeine stimulates the central nervous system, speeds up the heart, and acts as a diuretic. The nut and its preparations contain 1.5 percent caffeine and slight amounts of the asthma drug theobromine.

How to Use the Herb

Cola nuts are dried and powdered for medicinal use. Commission E approves these average daily doses: 2–6 grams of dried nut, 0.25–0.75 grams of cola extract, 2.5–7.5 grams of liquid extract, 10–30 grams of tincture.

Consumer Products Available

Cola nut powder is available in health food stores, sometimes in combination with other herbs, as a pick-me-up. (It's sometimes spelled "kola" on product labels.) Dried extracts and fluid extracts are sold, too, as is cola tincture.

Potential Dangers

Cola nut shouldn't be used by people with gastric or duodenal ulcers. The naturally occurring caffeine can increase the power of antidepressant drugs. Like other stimulants, it can cause sleeplessness, anxiety, and restlessness.

COMFREY HERB AND LEAF

Symphytum officinale

The value of comfrey, a small, hardy perennial with bell-shaped flowers, can be gleaned from other common names of the plant: bruisewort and knitbone. Known to the Greeks and the Romans, comfrey has a long—and recently controversial—place in the herbal pharmacy.

Potential Health Benefits

Commission E endorses the most-established use of comfrey leaf and comfrey root: the external use of comfrey ointments and creams to speed the healing of bruises, sprains, and pulled muscles and ligaments.

Scientific Evidence

Comfrey's efficacy at healing—it was favored in ancient times for treating battlefield wounds—is due to the chemical allantoin, which promotes cell reproduction and formation of new tissue. However, comfrey also contains toxic pyrrolizidine alkaloids (PAs), which have caused cancer in laboratory animals. The chemicals are most highly concentrated in the root; cancer risk comes from internal use of the root. Commission E endorses herb and leaf for external use only. Scientific articles published in the *American Journal of Medicine*, *Gastroenterology*, and the *British Medical Journal* in the 1980s and 1990s have documented the poisonous effects of PAs in comfrey root, even when the root is taken in tablets and teas. The root contains concentrations of PAs ten times higher than the leaves.

How to Use the Herb

Again: Commission E recommends comfrey leaf and herb for external use only. For the leaf: "Ointments and other preparations with 5–20 percent dried drug or equivalent preparations. The daily applied dose should not exceed 100 micrograms of pyrolizidine alkaloids." The same amounts obtain for comfrey root. The commission recommends "crushed leaf or root, extracts, and the pressed juice of the fresh plant for semi-solid preparations and poultices for external use."

Consumer Products Available

Ointments are available in health food stores and drugstores. Supplements for internal use sold in health food stores and elsewhere aren't recommended. The type of comfrey used commercially should be *S. officinale*, not any other species; they are less effective. Make sure the product label specifies *S. officinale*.

Potential Dangers

The potent cancer-causing agents in comfrey root rule out internal use. Even for external use, Commission E instructs pregnant women to consult a physician before using comfrey. It finds no known side effects or drug interactions. Comfrey use should be no longer than four to six weeks per year.

DANDELION

Taraxacum officinale

Everyone recognizes the sunny, spiky dandelion, and many consumers have sampled the drink made from dandelion root, which serves as a caffeine-free coffee substitute. Dandelion also has a healthful history going back centuries. Both the root and the above-ground plant are prized as medicine.

Potential Health Benefits

Dandelion is used to increase the flow of bile, aiding in the digestion of fats. It's also used as a diuretic, to restore appetite, and to calm an upset stomach.

Scientific Evidence

Ingredients include the bitter principles lactucopicrin (taraxacin), triterpenoids, and phytosterol. Dandelion leaves contain potassium, a mineral often lost when other diuretics are used. Dandelion's diuretic properties have been confirmed in animal studies, although it hasn't been extensively tested in controlled human studies.

How to Use the Herb

As a tea: 1 tablespoon of cut herb per cup of water, twice per day. As a decoction, 3–4 grams of cut or powdered herb per cup of water, boiled for 10 to 20 minutes, to extract more of the active principal than you can get from tea. As a tincture: 10–15 drops, taken 3 times per day.

Consumer Products Available

Dandelion is available in capsules and as dried flowers, root juice, powdered root, tinctures, and extracts in health food stores. Fresh, young leaves are nutritious and tasty in salads; older leaves are bitter-tasting.

Potential Dangers

Slight chance of heartburn. If you pick dandelions, try to make sure they come from a place that hasn't been sprayed with chemicals. There are no known drug interactions. Commission E warns that dandelion shouldn't be used by persons with obstructed bile ducts and cautions that those with gallstones should consult a physician before using it.

DEVIL'S CLAW ROOT

Harpagophytum procumbens

Devil's claw root gets its rather unpleasant name from its fruits, which reminded people of a claw-like hand. Fortunately, the medicinal effect of the plant, which is native to southern and central Africa, is pleasant indeed. The dried root is the medically useful part.

Potential Health Benefits

Devil's claw root stimulates the appetite, stimulates the production of bile for digesting fats, works to reduce inflammation, and has a mild ability to reduce pain.

Scientific Evidence

The herb contains bitter substances and a compound, harpagoside, which reduces inflammation and relieves pain. In a 1996 German study, 118 patients with lower back pain took 6 grams of dried devil's claw root with 50 milligrams of harpagoside. "Positive, though inconclusive, results in reducing or eliminating acute attacks of lower back pain were reported, promoting a call for more clinical studies," writes American herbal author Varro E. Tyler, Ph.D. In a 1976 German study, devil's claw was found to alleviate pain and to lower both high cholesterol and uric acid blood levels. However, Tyler notes, those results haven't been duplicated by subsequent studies. American author Steven B. Karch, M.D., suggests that "harpagoside both stimulates the release of, and is destroyed by, stomach acid," leading to a "highly variable rate of absorption." That, Karch writes, "may explain why clinical researchers have reported conflicting results."

How to Use the Herb

The powdered root can be taken in teas or supplements. Commission E's recommended daily dose for stimulating appetite is 1.5 grams. For other uses, the daily dose is 4.5 grams. Enteric-coated tablets may help boost the rate of absorption.

Consumer Products Available

Health food stores sell devil's claw root in capsules, tablets, tinctures, and as an ingredient in ointments.

Potential Dangers

Allergic reactions have occurred in persons with gastric and duodenal ulcers. People with gallstones should consult a physician before using devil's claw root.

DILL SEED

Anethum graveolens

Commonly used to pickle cucumbers, aromatic dill seeds come from an annual plant native to the Mediterranean region. Dill is related to parsley and carrots. Its seeds are actually the fruit produced at the top of dill's delicate, frond-like tops.

Potential Health Benefits

Dill is used to calm the stomach, aid digestion, and sweeten the breath. It also prevents the multiplication of bacteria in the intestinal tract.

Scientific Evidence

Dill seed, the dried fruit of the plant, contains an essential oil rich in carvone. The herb quiets spasms in the smooth muscles of the intestine, aiding digestion.

How to Use the Herb

Crushed or bruised dill seed can be made into a tea. Commission E's average daily doses are 3 grams from seed and 0.1–0.3 grams of the more powerful oil.

Consumer Products Available

Fresh and dried dill is available in health food stores and supermarkets, which often sell the whole plant, as well.

Potential Dangers

No major side effects or drug interactions. Dill can cause a skin rash and sensitivity to sunlight.

ECHINACEA

Echinacea purpurea, Echinacea pallida,
Echinacea angustifolia

Echinacea, a native of the central Great Plains of the United States
and a member of the daisy family, has become an herbal best-seller,
thanks to its reputation for knocking out colds and flu; this reputation is verified by Commission E. Three of the nine species of
echinacea are used medicinally, and two of those—*E. pallida* root
and *E. purpurea* herb—were evaluated by the commission. Native
Americans and others used the plant medicinally in the 19th century, but echinacea was eclipsed in North America until its popularity in Europe inspired a comeback on the cusp of the 21st century.

Potential Health Benefits

Clobbering colds and fighting flu. Anecdotal evidence that echinacea is effective in combating chronic fatigue syndrome, genital
herpes, and even ear infections wasn't addressed by the commission. American health writers have assigned broader uses to the
herb. Dr. Andrew Weil, in his book *Consumer Guide to Herbal
Medicine*, touts tincture of echinacea against sinusitis, tonsillitis, and
ear infections and recommends using it the day before and day after major dental work to prevent bacterial infections. Weil also recommends echinacea for travelers facing long airplane flights, with
their germ-laden, recycled air. Recent research in Germany suggests
that echinacea may be an effective fighter against yeast infections.

Scientific Evidence

Echinacea is so highly regarded that James A. Duke, Ph.D., a respected herbal researcher and writer, suggests that it could be use-

ful for patients with HIV/AIDS. Commission E disagrees, saying HIV/AIDS patients should not use echinacea. Since the herb stimulates the autoimmune system, it could make things worse for people whose immune systems are attacking the body, among them people with AIDS. Echinacea's wound-healing properties come from the fact that it has natural antibiotic properties; in fact, it was used as an antibiotic until sulfa and other new drugs came on the market in the 1930s. Researchers believe the herb stimulates production of interferon and disease-fighting T-cells. A 1984 study published in the journal *Infection and Immunology* concluded that echinacea produces formidable white blood cells (macrophages) that destroy germs. In a University of Munich study, echinacea produced 30 percent more infection-fighting T-cells than other drugs under review. In another German study, echinacea reduced the recurrence of vaginal yeast infections in a group of 203 women from 60 percent to 16 percent. All told, the research on echinacea is solid, extensive, and encouraging.

How to Use the Herb

Commission E recommends daily doses of tincture of ethanol corresponding to 900 milligrams for *E. pallida*. For *E. purpurea*, the commission recommends a daily dose of 6–9 milliliters of expressed juice, taken internally at the first signs of illness. For external use in a salve, Commission E recommends preparations with at least 15 percent expressed juice. Some health writers recommend echinacea tea, taken 3 to 4 times per day. Andrew Weil advises taking a full dose the day before an airline flight, the day of the flight, and for one or two days afterward.

Consumer Products Available

Echinacea is ubiquitous in health food stores, drugstores, and supermarkets. All three varieties used medically are available in tinctures,

The bewildering variety of echinacea products on the market can be decoded by keeping a few things in mind: Look for the Latin names on product labels, to make sure you're getting the right form of the plant; check to see what part of the plant was used, hopefully the leaf, as this is the most medicinally rich part; seriously consider buying single-plant preparations in preference to products that combine echinacea with other substances that may or may not have been tested.

As an example, Tom's of Maine sells a Natural Echinacea Liquid Extract, a single-plant product delivered in liquid form, which Commission E recommends. However, Tom's product label doesn't specify which form of echinacea is used in the product or what part of the plant was used. The label does include a toll-free telephone number, which is a good sign. By means of comparison, Dr. Art Ulene Herbal Formulas Standardized Echinacea Capsules contain 380 milligrams of the herb, a convenient dose, as just two or three pills a day would correspond to recommended dose levels; however, this product label, too, doesn't list the Latin name or specify what part of the plant was used. The label does have a toll-free telephone number, which is useful. Nature's Way Echinacea Capsules are also standardized at 380 milligrams, and the label additionally specifies the source: *Echinacea purpurea*, which was approved by Commission E. The label also states that the herb was organically grown and cites relevant state codes, although it doesn't specify which part of the plant was used. In the case of Nature's Bounty Herbal Harvest Echinacea with Goldenseal Root Herbal Supplement Capsules, the product combines echinacea with five other herbs. Even more amazingly, Ricola Herb Throat Lozenge Echinacea Green Tea, Sugar-Free counts no fewer than 11 herbs among its 20 ingredients. Commission E and prominent American health writers such as Andrew Weil, M.D., advise against making things too complicated. Last point: Many American herbal companies use *Echinacea augustifolia*; this apparently reflects differences in use between North America and Europe, and doesn't mean the products won't work, but there's not as much documentation backing them up. *Echinacea purpurea*, which the commission approved, has extensive research behind it.

teas, and capsules. Overharvesting has raised concerns that some commercial products contain precious little echinacea; read labels closely. Commission E didn't evaluate U.S. products that combine echinacea with the likes of goldenseal, zinc, and garlic. Cough drops and candies with echinacea are unlikely to contain enough of the herb to have medicinal value. Echinacea naturally makes the tongue tingle. If that doesn't happen, you're getting a low dose.

Potential Dangers

Commission E found no major side effects or interference with other drugs. However, the commission did recommend using echinacea for short-term use (not more than eight weeks), discontinuing use when symptoms of illness go away. Some North American herbalists recommend daily dosages of echinacea as an immune system booster, but this is controversial; long-term use could cause the body to build up a tolerance to this useful herb and render its therapeutic use ineffective. The commission recommends that people with AIDS/HIV stay away from echinacea. Many experts also warn against use of echinacea by persons with Type 1 diabetes, as well as those with multiple sclerosis. The injectable form of *echinacea purpurea* herb should not be used during pregnancy.

EUCALYPTUS LEAF AND OIL
Eucalyptus globulus

Native to Australia and now grown in many parts of the world, the eucalyptus tree is abundant in California and around the Mediterranean. The essential oil—strong but pleasant-smelling—is drawn from the leaves and is a prime ingredient in products such as Vicks VapoRub, Mentholatum Cherry Chest Rub, and Listerine mouthwash.

Potential Health Benefits

When it's inhaled, eucalyptus clears the lungs of mucous. It's used externally in ointments to ease rheumatic complaints by improving local circulation.

Scientific Evidence

The dried mature leaf from older trees contains essential oil, "which consists mainly of 1.8-cineol and tannins," according to Commission E. Oil is obtained by steam distillation of fresh leaves and branch tips and contains at least 70 percent of 1.8-cineol. In its various forms, eucalyptus is an exceptionally good decongestant. The U.S. Food and Drug Administration approves eucalyptus as a treatment for flu and colds. In his book *Plants That Heal*, Joel L. Swerdlow, Ph.D., refers to studies, which he doesn't name, that conclude that eucalyptus has the power to kill "some influenza viruses and some kinds of bacteria, making it a treatment for bronchitis."

How to Use the Herb

For internal use, the daily average dose from the leaf is 4–6 grams. For tincture, 3–9 grams. For external use, daily dose is 5–20 percent oil in semisolid preparations, 5–10 percent oil in aqueous-alcohol preparations, and several drops of the essential oil rubbed into the skin.

Consumer Products Available

Teas, tinctures, and ointments are sold in health food stores and drugstores.

Potential Dangers

Eucalyptus essential oil in its undiluted form shouldn't be applied to the faces of small children or swallowed by either children or adults. Persons with inflamed gastrointestinal tracts, inflamed bile ducts, or serious liver diseases shouldn't use eucalyptus preparations. Commission E suggests that eucalyptus leaf taken internally may weaken the potency of some drugs, but doesn't say which ones. Consult your health care provider before using eucalyptus leaf.

FENNEL OIL AND SEED

Foeniculum vulgare

A relative of parsley and carrots, fennel is a native of southern Europe, with yellow flowers and aromatic oil. It's a hardy perennial whose seed oil is used medicinally, as are the dried seeds themselves. It has a flavor similar to anise or licorice (see those entries).

Potential Health Benefits

Fennel is used chiefly to dispel flatulence, soothe spasms in the gastrointestinal tract, and loosen mucous from colds and bronchitis. Fennel honey and syrup are used to treat those symptoms in children. Moreover, crushed fennel seeds are used in an eyewash to treat conjunctivitis.

Scientific Evidence

Fennel oil, made from the dried, ripe fruits by steam distillation, contains up to 5 percent estragon, an estrogen-like substance; the dried seeds contain the same amount of estragon. According to Beth Ann Petro Roybal and Gayle Skowronski's book *Sex Herbs*, fennel may increase the sex drive in women. Fennel seeds and oil also contain anethole and fenchone, which, Commission E notes, have been shown in laboratory tests to break down secretions in the respiratory tract.

How to Use the Herb

For fennel oil, the daily dose is 0.1–0.6 milliliters (2–12 drops). For fennel honey and syrup standardization to 0.5 grams of fennel oil, 10–20 grams. For fennel seed, 5–7 grams of the herb, and

5.0–7.5 grams of tincture. Crushed or ground fennel can be made into a tea: 1–2 teaspoonfuls steeped for 10 minutes and taken up to 3 times per day is a common dose.

Consumer Products Available

Fresh fennel is sold in health food stores, herb shops, and supermarkets. Seed capsules and tinctures are available in health food stores and drugstores.

Potential Dangers

Pregnant women shouldn't use fennel. Fennel should also not be given to infants or toddlers. Diabetics should check the sugar content of fennel honey and syrup. Fennel oil preparations shouldn't be used for more than two weeks.

Fenugreek Seed

Trigonella foenum-graecum

Fenugreek (from the Latin for "Greek hay") is native to Mediterranean countries and is a popular additive in horse rations. It's good for people, too. Fenugreek flavors Indian curries and has a range of modern and traditional medical uses, several of which were validated by Commission E.

Potential Health Benefits

Fenugreek, taken internally, is used to stimulate the appetite. Applied externally, it's used in poultices for local inflammation. Some writers credit fenugreek with increasing milk production for nursing mothers, as well as elevating the sex drive in women—points not addressed by Commission E.

Scientific Evidence

The ripe, dried seed contains bitter principles and mucilage that, when mixed with water, produces a paste useful in poultices. Commission E also found that fenugreek is secretolytic: that is, it breaks down secretions in the lungs, and is a mild antiseptic, as well. The *PDR Family Guide to Natural Medicines & Healing Therapies* reports that "Researchers have been unable to pinpoint the active ingredient in the herb." Health writer Steven B. Karch, M.D., writes that an amino acid in fenugreek, 4-hydroxyisoleucine, "increases glucose-induced insulin from the pancreas." While Commission E didn't address fenugreek's use as a treatment for diabetes, Karch comments: "Claims about treating diabetes [with fenugreek] appear to have a basis in fact." In a 1996 study published in *Phytotherapy Research*, scientists found that fenugreek seed triggered a

14 percent reduction in serum cholesterol levels in 60 non-insulin-dependent diabetics in a 24-week trial.

How to Use the Herb

For internal use, the daily dose is 6 grams of the seed. For external use, liniments, ointments, gels, emulsions, and oils can be used. Fenugreek can also be steamed an inhaled, by putting 50 grams of powdered herb into ¼ liter of water.

Consumer Products Available

Health food stores sell fenugreek seeds and seed capsules.

Potential Dangers

Fenugreek has no known drug interactions, but it can produce skin irritation from repeated external use. Commission E reports no other major side effects. Some authors caution pregnant women to limit their use of fenugreek or avoid it in medicinal doses entirely. Please check with your obstetrician before using it.

FLAXSEED

Linum usitatissimun

You probably use flaxseed even if you don't know it. Fiber made from this plant's stems are spun into linen. The seeds are pressed to produce linseed oil. A slender plant with delicate blue flowers, flax is widely cultivated. The small brown seeds and their oil are also used medicinally.

Potential Health Benefits

Flaxseed is used to treat chronic constipation, irritable colon, diverticulitis, and colons damaged by abusing commercial laxatives. Assertions by researchers that flaxseed (or linseed oil) protects against some cancers and eases menstrual discomfort weren't addressed by Commission E. Flax preparations can soothe irritations when rubbed on the skin.

Scientific Evidence

Flaxseed contains fiber and fatty oil with 52–76 percent linolenic acid esters. A University of Toronto study found that flaxseed fed to animals for seven weeks reduced the size of tumors by more than half. The same study found that an ingredient in flaxseed, called lignan, seemed to block the creation of new tumors. According to the *Prevention* magazine book *Nature's Medicines*, "Many plants have some lignan, but flaxseed has at least 75 times more than almost any other plant."

How to Use the Herb

As cracked seeds or mush, taken internally. As flaxseed flour for a moist-heat compress applied externally. For internal use, take 1 tablespoon of whole or bruised seed with 150 milliliters of water 2 to 3 times per day, with meals. Or 2–3 tablespoonfuls of milled flaxseed for mush. For external use, 30–50 grams of flaxseed flour for a moist-heat compress.

Consumer Products Available

Flaxseeds and linseed oil are sold in health food stores and supermarkets, as are capsules with linseed oil. The oil, however, lacks the seeds' fiber. Commission E endorses seed.

Potential Dangers

The absorption of drugs could be weakened by using flaxseed.

GARLIC

Allium sativum

Ah, the monarch of herbs. Garlic has been used to treat a staggeringly large variety of ills, in virtually every culture, for at least 5,000 years. Believed to be native to central Asia, garlic was dubbed "the stinking rose" by the Romans. A relative of onions, shallots, chives, and leeks, garlic—more specifically, the cloves from garlic bulbs, the underground part of the plant—is a perennial in the herbal hall of fame. Garlic is a member of the lily family.

Potential Health Benefits

Commission E endorses garlic as a treatment for age-related vascular changes and for lowering high cholesterol. Garlic has antibiotic qualities and has traditionally been used to disinfect wounds. Folklore around the world credits garlic for helping to lower high blood pressure, thus providing a measure of protection against heart attacks and strokes.

Scientific Evidence

Garlic is very high in the sulfur compounds also used in commercial high blood pressure medications. Garlic contains compounds that thin the blood and slow clotting. Many studies attribute garlic's health benefits to allicin, which gives the plant its strong "garlic" smell. A study at the University of California–Irvine found an 11-percent reduction in cholesterol levels among men who took garlic and fish oil supplements; men taking a placebo showed no significant reduction. A 1998 study reported in the *Harvard Health Letter* found no reduction of fat-soluble lipids in a clinical trial. However, garlic has scored high marks in most of the more than

2,000 studies of the herb done worldwide, and shows a wide range of benefits. In a 1994 study of women in Iowa, garlic prompted a significant reduction in colon cancer rates. In the book *Garlic: The Science and Therapeutic Application of Allium Sativum and Related Species*, editors Heinrich P. Koch, Ph.D., and Larry D. Lawson, Ph.D., reviewed 40 clinical trials, finding that garlic lowered triglycerides, which carry fat in the blood, by a healthy average of 13 percent.

How to Use the Herb

Garlic can be eaten raw, provided that you find it digestible and can tolerate garlic breath (parsley is traditionally paired with garlic as a breath-freshener) or cooked as part of your meals. Commission E recommends a daily dose of 400 milligrams, the equivalent of 1 clove. Some garlic fans believe that cooking weakens garlic's health benefits, a point not addressed by the commission.

Consumer Products Available

Whole garlic bulbs, garlic powder, and minced garlic cloves in oil are widely available in health food stores and supermarkets. Garlic supplements are sold in health food stores, drugstores, and supermarkets as dried and deodorized tablets or capsules containing garlic oil (the ingredient allicin, however, is inactive in oil). Fresh-cut garlic appears to be the most medicinally useful form of the herb.

Potential Dangers

Dragon breath, of course, and sometimes indigestion. Generally, garlic is very safe. It has no serious side effects or known adverse reactions with other drugs, although some experts advise limiting garlic intake if you're also taking anticoagulant medications.

POWER 8 HERB
GARLIC

If you can't use fresh garlic, and are trying to sort out the garlic supplements on the market, here are a couple of things to keep in mind: Look for supplements with labels that tell you that the product has standardized amounts of allicin, and check the amount of garlic in each dose. Very high doses might be a waste of money; very low ones could mean you'll have to take repeated doses to get to recommended levels. For example, GNC Herbal Plus Concentrated Garlic Softgel Capsules come in whopping 1,000 milligram doses; one pill is 2½ times Commission E's recommended dose for the whole day. GNC also sells GNC Natural Brand Odorless Garlic Tablets at 270 milligrams each, which may be more manageable and efficient, although the company recommends taking 2–4 tablets per day, which is a lot of garlic. Nature Made High Potency Garlic Oil Softgels contain oil equivalent to 1,500 milligrams of garlic. With the company's suggested doses of 4 per day, you'd be getting 15 times Commission E's recommended amount! Individuals vary, but some people might also have difficulty digesting that much.

GINGER

Zingiber officinale

Originating in Southeast Asia, ginger has long been used in cooking and medicine in the ancient cultures of India and China. Europeans and North Americans adapted ginger to flavor ginger ale, gingerbread, and other edibles. The medically useful parts of ginger, a perennial tropical plant, are identified by Commission E as "the peeled, finger-long, fresh and dried rhizome of *Zingiberis rhizoma*." Rhizomes are underground stems that resemble roots.

Potential Health Benefits

Commission E endorses ginger as an antidote for dyspepsia—upset stomach—and as a preventative for motion sickness. Some traditional uses in Asian medicine, such as treatment for asthma and earache, weren't evaluated.

Scientific Evidence

Ginger is an antiemetic—that is, it prevents vomiting and dispels nausea. It also stimulates secretion of saliva and gastric juices, aiding digestion. Ginger's anti-nausea components are gingerol and shogaol. A double-blind study published in the British journal *Lancet* in 1982 found that 940 milligrams of powdered ginger were more effective than 100 milligrams of dimenhydrate (Dramamine); the test was done on 36 college students considered susceptible to motion sickness. Most studies since then have confirmed ginger's value against motion sickness. In a 1998 U.S. study that combined ginger with vitamin B_6 supplements and the use of acupressure, the combination reduced nausea and vomiting during pregnancy. Ginger is apparently good for that especially unpleasant form of motion sickness, seasickness, too. A 1988 Danish study of 80 Danish teenaged cadets found that 1,000 milligrams of powdered ginger was more effective than a placebo in combating seasickness.

How to Use the Herb

Fresh or dried ginger root in soups, rice, or stir-fry dishes add zest. Medicinal doses are set by Commission E at 2–4 grams per day (up to 1 teaspoonful) in the form of chopped rhizome or dry extract. To make ginger tea, pour boiling water over 0.5–1.0 grams of powdered ginger (¼ teaspoonful) and steep for 5 minutes.

Consumer Products Available

Fresh, chopped, and powdered ginger is available in groceries, especially in Asian neighborhoods, and as supplements in health food stores.

Potential Dangers

According to Commission E, ginger shouldn't be used by people with gallstones or during pregnancy—although the pregnancy warning is challenged by some, including the American Botanic Council, an industry trade group, which considers ginger safe during pregnancy. Ginger has no known negative interactions with other drugs.

GINKGO BILOBA LEAF

Ginkgo biloba

Ginkgo has been dubbed the memory tree. The oldest living tree species on Earth, it was around in the time of the dinosaurs, and is native to northeast Asia. Some ginkgo trees live for up to 1,000 years, and its toughness makes it a good choice for lining the streets of polluted cities. Medically, ginkgo is used to prevent or slow memory loss associated with aging, Alzheimer's disease, and other causes. The leaves are the most medically useful part of the tree, and the safest, as the fruit and seeds are high in toxins.

Potential Health Benefits

Prime benefits of ginkgo, according to Commission E, which assessed the standardized dry extract of green, fan-shaped ginkgo leaves, include: improving memory and learning capacity; strengthening blood flow to the brain; treating vertigo; zapping destructive free radicals in the blood; and reducing swelling and lesions in the retina of the eye. In short, ginkgo is great for the circulation. In Germany, it's used to treat memory loss and dementia. Commission E also found ginkgo useful for treating some forms of tinnitus (ringing in the ear). With annual sales topping $500 million, ginkgo is Europe's best-selling herbal drug.

Scientific Evidence

Commission E and other researchers attribute ginkgo's medical powers to its ability to increase blood flow to the brain and extremities such as hands and feet. Active chemicals in ginkgo, called ginkgolides, have a blood-thinning effect. Dozens of clinical studies of GBE extract—the standardized European ginkgo drug—

have been published in Europe, especially Germany. A U.S. study of 202 patients with dementia, published in 1997 in the *Journal of the American Medical Association*, concluded that daily doses of 120 milligrams of GBE strengthened and in some cases improved the mental functions of people who took it for up to one year.

How to Use the Herb

Commission E recommends daily doses of 120–240 milligrams of dry ginkgo extract in 2 or 3 divided doses to combat memory loss. For vertigo and tinnitus, the daily dose is 120–160 milligrams of dry extract, also in 2 or 3 divided daily doses. Several herbal authorities caution that teas made from ginkgo leaves, a standby of traditional Chinese medicine, are too weak to do much medicinally.

Consumer Products Available

Ginkgo biloba is available in tablets and capsules in health food stores, drugstores, and supermarkets. Supplements should contain an extract of 24 percent flavone glycosides and 6 percent ginkgolides; this is the standard formula used in scientific studies. In the U.S., common brands of European-standard supplements are sold under the names Ginkgold and Ginkoba.

Potential Dangers

The commission found no lethal level of overdoses or side effects but doesn't recommend using ginkgo for longer than eight weeks. Ginkgo shouldn't be used if you're taking blood-thinners, including aspirin.

When buying products containing this very popular herb, keep several things in mind. First, look for products that specify use of the leaf, which is the most medically active part of the ginkgo tree. Second, check to see if the product label specifies that the product contains an extract of 24 percent flavone glycosides and 6 percent ginkgolides, the standard formula used in scientific studies. Third, check warning labels; they should tell people using blood-thinners—including aspirin—to steer clear of ginkgo. Unless things have changed since I wrote this, however, the manufacturers probably won't point out this important information. When I reviewed seven ginkgo products for this book, all advised keeping supplements out of the reach of children, which is, of course, important and correct, but none cited aspirin use.

A good example of a supplement formulated to recommended levels is Centrum Naturals, which specifies that the product comes from leaves, is standardized to "24/6" (see above), and, at 60 milligrams taken twice a day, clocks in at the acceptably lower end of Commission E's recommended daily amount. Drugstore.com Ginkgo Biloba Caplets are also within the commission's range, with 60 milligrams taken three times a day, and use the "24/6" formulation (see paragraph one in this box), but don't specify that the product came from the leaf. Nature's Bounty Herbal Harvest Ginkgo Biloba Herbal Supplement has the same specifications as Drugstore.com's product and, similarly, doesn't specify use of the leaf. Some products may be "busier" and more complex than they need to be. GNC Herbal Plus Standardized Ginkgo Biloba Herbal Supplements include two other herbs, on the apparent assumption that more is better—which isn't always true. One-a-Day Memory & Concentration, which, the manufacturer states, "goes beyond just Ginkgo biloba," includes the mineral choline and B-vitamins. That combination may be fine, but its efficacy is unproven.

GINSENG
Panax ginseng

Ginseng—from the Chinese words for "man root," because the root resembles the shape of the human body—springs from the forest primeval. Originally harvested in the wild in North America and East Asia, it was used in traditional Asian medicine as a panacea: a cure-all. Today, ginseng is grown commercially, notably in Wisconsin, for export to Asia and is used in many parts of the world as a tonic.

Potential Health Benefits

Commission E tested the dried root of *Panax ginseng*, the form of the herb native to Asia. Researchers endorsed ginseng's value as a "tonic for invigoration and fortification in times of fatigue and debility, and declining work and concentration, also during convalescence." In short, it's a pick-me-up and stress-buster. Some health practitioners employ ginseng to treat chronic fatigue syndrome and depression.

Scientific Evidence

Ginseng's pharmacological actions are attributed to panaxosides and ginsenosides, which are thought to stimulate the central nervous system. These substances are present in all three varieties of ginseng: *Panax ginseng* (Asian ginseng), *Panax quinquefolius* (American ginseng), and *Eleutherococcus senticosus* (Siberian ginseng, a cousin of the other two).

POWER 8 HERB
GINSENG

If you're shopping for ginseng supplements, not ginseng root itself, make sure that the label specifies the product is standardized to at least 4 percent ginsenocides. The preferred form of ginseng approved by Commission E is *Panax ginseng*. Look for this Latin name on the label. Other forms are also sold. Nature's Herbs Siberian Ginseng Powder Herb Capsules, for example, contain Siberian ginseng, a relative of *Panax* approved by Commission E as a tonic but not as highly valued. Drugstore.com Ginseng Caplets contain *Panax* and are standardized to 7 percent ginsenocides, which is good, but contain only 100 milligrams of ginseng. To get Commission E's recommended dose, you'll have to take 10 to 20 a day. Ginseng Gold Concentrated Ginseng Extract for Tea says "Korean ginseng" on the label but doesn't give the Latin name, which would be more scientifically specific, and furthermore contains alcohol and sugars to make the bitter-tasting ginseng palatable. Ginseng Gold Korean Ginseng & Royal Jelly Capsules combine the herb with royal jelly, a substance made for queen bees by worker bees. The jelly has an extravagant reputation in some health circles but wasn't studied by Commission E, either in combination with ginseng or otherwise.

How to Use the Herb

You can chew bits of the whole root, although it's bitter-tasting, or take ginseng in tablets, in sweetened teas, as a powdered root, or in a tincture. Commission E used cut root for teas and powders and recommends 1–2 grams per day.

Consumer Products Available

Health food stores, supermarkets, and drugstores stock a wide range of commercial preparations; the root can be found in health food stores and herb shops, especially in Chinese neighborhoods. Supplements should contain 7 percent ginsenocides, a standard level. Candies, soft drinks, and other snacks fortified with ginseng are unlikely to have enough ginseng to be medically active.

Potential Dangers

Ginseng can overstimulate the central nervous system, causing anxiety, insomnia, diarrhea, and high blood pressure. Commission E found no known interactions with other drugs, but advises discontinuing use after three months, commenting that "a repeated course is feasible." Some health practitioners say heart patients shouldn't use ginseng.

GOLDENROD

Solidago species

Goldenrod (not to be confused with goldenseal) has rod-like stems and bright yellow leaves. The above-ground parts of the plant are gathered during flowering season. Commission E tested both European goldenrod (*virgaureae*) and other forms (*herba*), and didn't differentiate between them in its evaluation.

Potential Health Benefits

Goldenrod is a diuretic, flushing out the urinary tract, which makes the herb valuable for treating urinary tract infection. It's also used to treat kidney and bladder stones.

Scientific Evidence

Commission E found that the herb has mild antispasmotic qualities and can help prevent inflammation of the urinary tract. Its recommendations are drawn from goldenrod's long history of use in German medicine.

How to Use the Herb

The daily dose is 6–12 grams of the dried herb, the equivalent of 2–4 teaspoonfuls. Be sure to take it with lots of water. Goldenrod tea can be made by taking 3–5 grams (1–2 teaspoonfuls) of crushed herb, steeping for 15 minutes in hot water, and drinking it 2 to 4 times per day between meals.

Consumer Products Available

Health food stores sell dried goldenrod, along with teas, liquid extracts, and tinctures.

Potential Dangers

Goldenrod shouldn't be used if you have edema (swelling) from heart or kidney conditions. It has no known interactions with other drugs.

HARONGA BARK AND LEAF

Haronga madagascariensis

An evergreen tree native to East Africa, the haronga is found throughout tropical Africa. The bark and leaf of the plant are used medicinally after being stripped from the tree and air-dried.

Potential Health Benefits

Haronga can settle an upset stomach. It's also used to treat mild insufficiencies of enzymes from the pancreas, the better to digest protein and fat.

Scientific Evidence

Haronga stimulates the digestive juices, stimulates the pancreas, stimulates the liver to increase bile production, and increases production of the gastrointestinal hormone cholecystokinin, which helps gallbladder function. It hasn't yet been studied extensively in controlled clinical trials, although *The PDR Family Guide to Natural Medicines & Healing Therapies*, without citing sources, reports that the bark and leaf "have exhibited a protective effect on the liver" in animal tests.

How to Use the Herb

Haronga is taken as an extract. Average daily dosage is 7.5–15.0 milligrams. Don't use longer than two months.

Consumer Products Available

Health food stores sell haronga extract, although it's not as widely available in the United States as many herbs.

Potential Dangers

Persons who shouldn't use haronga at all include: people with acute pancreatitis, severe liver disorders, gallstones, and obstruction of the bile ducts. Overdoses can make you sensitive to sunlight.

HAWTHORN LEAF WITH FLOWER

Crataegus monogyna

Hawthorn is a small, thorny bush traditionally regarded in Europe as a heart tonic. Also known as mayflower, it's related to the apple tree and the peach tree, and is grown in hedgerows. It produces white, pink, and red flowers and red fruits, called haws, that look like tiny red apples.

Potential Health Benefits

Hawthorn is a preventative medicine and long-term treatment for painful angina attacks. Only the hawthorn leaf with flowers is approved by Commission E, which hasn't endorsed other forms of hawthorn, such as the fruit.

Scientific Evidence

Hawthorn dilates blood vessels, strengthening and speeding up the heartbeat. It contains flavonoids, which some researchers credit with helping to maintain a regular heartbeat, and oligomeric proanthocyanidins (OPCs), active principles credited by researchers with having sedative effects. A German study of 78 people with congestive heart failure showed that patients taking 600 milligrams of hawthorn extract per day lowered their blood pressure and raised their performance on a stationary bicycle. Other studies, most of them conducted in Europe, have drawn similarly encouraging conclusions, prompting American herbal authority Varro E. Tyler, Ph.D., to write: "[more] studies are urgently needed for a drug as potentially valuable as this one."

How to Use the Herb

Commission E favors a water-ethanol extract of 160–900 milligrams with defined flavonoid or proanthocyanidin content in "2 or 3 individual doses." It recommends using the herb for a minimum of six weeks, not citing a maximum term.

Consumer Products Available

Health food stores and drugstores sell hawthorn tinctures, extracts, powders, capsules, and fresh and dried herb.

Potential Dangers

Commission E emphasizes that patients with known or suspected heart disease absolutely must consult a physician, and not self-medicate. European clinicians recommend hawthorn as a long-term treatment, not for immediate, acute angina. It has no known drug interactions, contraindications, or side effects.

Hops

Humulus lupulus

This famed flavoring agent for beer is a climbing vine with green, cone-shaped flowers; it's the dried cones of the female flowers that are used in brewing, and in medicine. Hops are related to hemp and marijuana, but don't produce a high when they're smoked.

Potential Health Benefits

Hops are recommended to curb restlessness and anxiety and to treat sleep disturbances by Commission E, which also endorses hops for use as a sedative. Traditionally, pillows stuffed with hops have been used by people with insomnia.

Scientific Evidence

Hops contain bitter principles called humulene and lupulene (which give the sharp taste to English beers called bitters) and 2-methyl-3-butne-2-01, a chemical with sedative properties. The active principle of hops is located in a yellow powder, called lupulin, that surrounds the seed of the fruit. A 1996 German double-blind study found hops as effective as the drug Rohypnol when it comes to inducing sleep, with fewer side effects. Hops also contain phyto-estrogens, substances similar to estrogen, which may help prevent coronary disease and osteoporosis, although Commission E didn't address these larger possible effects of hops.

How to Use the Herb

A six-pack a day keeps . . . just kidding. Actually, sober-minded Commission E recommends the use of cut, powdered hops or extract in a single dose of 0.5 grams. If drops are used, 1 or 2 drops are the right amount. Hop tea can be made by pouring boiling water over a heaping teaspoonful of the ground herb and steeping for 10–15 minutes.

Consumer Products Available

Hops are sold in health food stores and herb shops as drops, dried, or fresh herb and extract.

Potential Dangers

The fresh plant can irritate the skin. Otherwise, hops get a clean bill of health. There are no known drug interactions, contraindications, or side effects.

HOREHOUND HERB

Marrubium vulgare

Horehound—also known as houndbane—is native to the Mediterranean region and is one of the bitter herbs consumed at Jewish Passover feasts. It's a bitter member of the mint family, with white, downy leaves. Commission E approved use of the above-ground parts of the plant, both fresh and dried.

Potential Health Benefits

Horehound is approved to treat loss of appetite, bloating, and flatulence. Traditionally, horehound has also been used as an expectorant and a treatment for bronchial coughs. In 1989, the United States banned horehound from cough medicines, saying it was ineffective. Commission E doesn't comment on horehound in cough remedies.

Scientific Evidence

Horehound contains bitter principles and tannins. It also contains marrubinic acid, which stimulates the liver to increase production of bile used by the body to digest fats. In a 1959 study, published in *Planta Medica*, marrubinic acid stimulated the production of bile, which speeds digestion, in rats. In a 1996 study, a horehound alcoholic extract reduced smooth-muscle spasms of the intestinal tract, lending credence to horehound's reputation as a digestive aid.

How to Use the Herb

Dried herb and freshly expressed juice are endorsed for internal use. The daily dosages are 4.5 grams of the herb and 2–6 tablespoonfuls of juice. *The PDR Family Guide to Natural Medicines & Healing Therapies* additionally recommends ½ tablespoonful of liquid extract 3 times per day, or up to 3 cups of tea per day.

Consumer Products Available

Horehound is available in health food stores in teas, extracts, tinctures, and juice.

Potential Dangers

There are no known contraindications, drug interactions, or side effects, according to Commission E, but some herbal authors advise against its use by heart patients.

HORSE CHESTNUT SEED

Aesculus hippocastanum

Widely grown in southeastern Europe, the European version of horse chestnut is a tall tree, called horse chestnut because the crushed nut is added to horse feed. The American variety is common in Ohio, where it's called buckeye. The seeds are peeled, mashed, and pulped for medical use.

Potential Health Benefits

Extract from the seed was reviewed and approved by Commission E for chronic venous insufficiency and pathological conditions of the veins of the legs. Horse chestnut seed can stop swelling of the legs, cramps in the calves, and pain and feeling of heaviness in the legs. (The flowers, bark, and other plant parts weren't specifically endorsed.)

Scientific Evidence

The active ingredient in horse chestnut seed is aescin (also spelled escin). It tightens up the walls of the capillaries, helping to prevent blood leakage, and reduces the activity of lyposomal enzymes implicated in causing problems in the veins of the legs. In a 1996 German study, test subjects with varicose veins who took 50 milligrams of aescin per day achieved as much reduction in their legs as people wearing compression stockings who didn't take supplements.

How to Use the Herb

The daily dose is 100 milligrams of aescin, corresponding to 250.0–312.5 milligrams of extract. Take it twice per day in delayed-release form.

Consumer Products Available

Health food stores sell standardized capsules and tinctures.

Potential Dangers

The PDR Family Guide to Natural Medicines & Healing Therapies cautions that high doses can cause enlarged pupils, unconsciousness, and other alarming conditions. *Prevention* magazine's book *Nature's Medicines* warns that horse chestnut seeds can interfere with the blood-thinner wafarin (Coumadin). Traditionally, the unprocessed nut has been considered toxic.

However, Commission E finds no known contraindications or drug interactions. It concludes that "pruritis, nausea and gastric complaints may occur in isolated cases after oral intake."

Horseradish

Armoracia rusticana

Horseradish is a perennial herb native to Russia that's now widely grown. One of the five bitter herbs of the Jewish Passover feast, horseradish is a member of the mustard family. The white, fleshy root is the part used medicinally, and is the source of the fiery wasabi of Japanese cuisine.

Potential Health Benefits

Horseradish loosens catarrhs of the upper respiratory tract when used either internally or externally. Used internally, it's also a treatment for urinary tract infection. Used externally, it can soothe minor muscle aches and pains.

Scientific Evidence

The herb contains mustard oil and mustard oil glycodiden. It kills or limits the growth of bacteria and can bring increased concentration of blood when applied to the skin. In animal studies, horseradish has relieved muscle spasms.

How to Use the Herb

Watch out: Hot! Used at the recommended doses, however, horseradish can do more than torch the inside of your mouth. For internal use, the average daily dose is 20 grams of fresh root or equivalent preparation. For external use, preparations with a minimum 2 percent mustard oil.

Consumer Products Available

Health food stores and supermarkets sell fresh and dried, cut and ground horseradish. Pressed juice is sometimes sold in stores.

Potential Dangers

Burning of the mouth and tongue, upset stomach. Persons with ulcers and kidney maladies shouldn't use horseradish, nor should it be given to children under four.

HORSETAIL HERB

Equisetum arvense

Looking like rushes or bamboo, the horsetail herb is also known as horse willow, toadpipe, and bottle brush. It's a perennial flowerless plant whose medicinal properties are found in the hollow, jointed stems.

Potential Health Benefits

Horsetail flushes fluid from the body and is a mild diuretic. It's useful for speeding slowly healing wounds, in combination with other therapies. It also has the power to help knock out bacterial and inflammatory diseases of the lower urinary tract and flush out kidney and bladder stones.

Scientific Evidence

The fresh or dried, green stems of horsetail, collected in summer, contain silicic acid and flavonoids. Its diuretic quality comes from the chemical ingredient equisetonin. German health authorities say that horsetail's silica and silicic acid doesn't test out as a useful treatment for bleeding tubercular lesions—contrary to some advocates of the herb.

How to Use the Herb

Internally, use powdered herb for infusions, taken orally in an average daily dose of 6 grams. Externally use 10 grams of powdered herb in 1 liter of water for compresses. If you take horsetail internally, drink plenty of water.

Consumer Products Available

Health food stores and drugstores sell powdered capsules and tablets.

Potential Dangers

Don't use horsetail if you have swelling caused by heart or kidney disease. There are no known drug interactions or side effects, according to Commission E.

JUNIPER BERRY

Juniperus communis

If you like gin, you like juniper. Juniper berries flavor gin. The cone-like berries are blue or red and grow on aromatic evergreen shrubs and trees closely related to cedar. Oil from the berries is used for flavoring, and for medicine.

Potential Health Benefits

Commission E endorses juniper berries for treating dyspepsia; that is, they settle the stomach. Juniper also helps restore flagging appetite. Because of its flushing, diuretic action, juniper is used to treat kidney and bladder stones.

Scientific Evidence

Juniper berries are steamed to produce volatile oil, which comprises about 1 percent of the dried herb. The oil contains terpineol 4-01, which gives juniper its diuretic power. Berries also contain tannins, sugars, flavonoid glycosides, and resin- and wax-containing compounds. Although it has long been favored in European folk medicine, controlled scientific studies aren't plentiful. American herbal authority Varro E. Tyler, Ph.D., concludes that "additional research on this ancient herbal remedy is certainly warranted."

How to Use the Herb

The daily dose is up to 10 grams of the dried berries, corresponding to 20–100 milligrams of the essential oil. Whole, crushed, or powdered herb can be used for infusions or decoctions, as can tinctures taken orally.

Consumer Products Available

Juniper berries, oil, tincture, syrup, and extract are sold at health food stores and herb shops.

Potential Dangers

Don't use for more than six weeks. Pregnant women and persons with inflamed kidneys shouldn't use juniper berry.

KAVA KAVA

Piper methysticum

Hugely popular as a ceremonial and social drink in Polynesian societies, kava—or kava kava, as it's popularly known—is valued medically as well as socially. The root of the kava, a large, flowering tropical shrub and member of the pepper family, is the medicinal part. Kava kava can grow more than ten feet high in its native region, the South Pacific.

Potential Health Benefits

The dried rhizomes of kava kava are endorsed by Commission E for treating nervous anxiety, stress, and restlessness. In short, kava kava is a feel-good herb, a natural Valium. Its heart-shaped leaves, too, are chewed in Polynesia, also to calm people down. Used in medicinal doses, kava kava is calming without being intoxicating or clouding the mind. In Germany, commercial kava drugs are sold under the names Kavasporal and Laitan, and in Great Britain consumers know it as Potter's Antigian Tablets.

Scientific Evidence

Kavalactones, a cluster of chemicals found in kava root, are believed to be the source of the feeling of well-being that kava induces. The herb also includes the pain-relieving chemicals dihydrokawain and dromethysticin. Researchers in clinical trials have found that an extract containing all of kava's ingredients worked better than a pure kavalactone extract. In a German study of 101 patients, those taking kava kava reported significantly less anxiety than those taking a placebo. Researchers have found that kava affects the lower central nervous system, not the brain—unlike prescription tranquilizers, which explains how the latter can cloud thinking. In matchups with prescription drugs in European trials, kava kava has frequently worked just as well, and has nearly always shown fewer side effects.

How to Use the Herb

Commission E recommends dried rhizomes in daily doses of 60–120 milligrams of kava-pyrones, or in supplements standardized to 70 percent kavalactones.

Consumer Products Available

Health food stores sell dried kava, as well as capsules, extracts, and tinctures. Supplements should be standardized to 70 percent kava-lactones.

Potential Dangers

Pregnant women, nursing mothers, or people who are clinically depressed shouldn't use kava kava. Kava kava can increase the potency of alcohol, barbiturates, and other drugs, although kava itself isn't addictive. With overdose or prolonged use, yellowed skin can result, and fingernails can become discolored. Don't use for more than three months without a physician's supervision.

LAVENDER FLOWER

Lavandula angustifolia

This fragrant member of the mint family is well-known for adding its natural perfume to the garden and to sachets, linens, and baths. The aromatic essential oil is derived from the plant's spiky, pale-purple flowers, which are also the part of the plant reviewed by Commission E.

Potential Health Benefits

Internally, lavender is used to lighten mood disturbances such as restlessness, end insomnia, dispel gas, and calm the stomach. Externally, it's used to perfume the bath and treat functional circulatory disorders.

Scientific Evidence

Lavender contains at least 1.5 percent essential oil, which includes camphor and "about 12 percent tannins unique to the family *Laamiaacea*," according to the commission. Lavender has been shown to work well against insomnia, among test subjects who sniffed fragrance of lavender. Scientific studies of more ambitious uses of lavender are scant. American herbal author Steven B. Karch, M.D., observes: "There has been pathetically little modern research on this herb. Laboratory studies suggest it is both antimicrobial and antifungal. Very limited clinical trials with inhalation suggest some improvement in chronic bronchitis. For many centuries, the essential oil has been recommended as an antiseptic, but clinical trials have never been undertaken."

How to Use the Herb

Internally, as a tea, use 1–2 teaspoonfuls of dried flower per cup of water; with lavender oil, put 1–4 drops on a sugar cube. Externally, as a bath additive, sprinkle anywhere from 20 to 100 grams of dried flowers in the water.

Consumer Products Available

Extracts, dried flowers, essential oil, and tinctures are sold in health food stores, drugstores, herb shops, and supermarkets.

Potential Dangers

High amounts of lavender may make you drowsier than you wanted or expected. A few people get a skin rash from the essential oil. Otherwise, there are no known side effects, contraindications, or drug interactions.

LEMON BALM

Melissa officinalis

The fragrant and pretty lemon balm, a form of mint, is one of the good guys of the herb garden and pantry. Modern herbalists use the plant's green leaves medicinally, as the ancient Romans did. Native to the eastern Mediterranean, lemon balm is cultivated widely and known under a variety of names, including melissa, sweet balm, sweet mary, and cure-all.

Potential Health Benefits

Lemon balm lives up to its name; it's a balm for a nervous stomach and a treatment for sleep disorders.

Scientific Evidence

Lemon balm leaves contain terpenes, which are tranquilizing agents, plus bitter principles and flavonoids according to Commission E. In addition to its sedative effects, lemon balm reduces flatulence. The herb's lemon smell comes from citronella, which is also present in lemons and lemongrass. Animal studies have shown antibacterial, antitumor, and antiviral effects. These results haven't been obtained in humans, however, where controlled studies of lemon balm are few in number.

How to Use the Herb

Fresh leaves and dry extracts make a refreshing tea. Use 1.5–4.5 grams of dried leaves. Or pour boiling water over a sprig of fresh leaves and steep for several minutes for a lovely, lemon-scented tea.

Consumer Products Available

Loose and bagged teas from the dried leaves are sold in health food stores and supermarkets, as are fresh plants and liquid and dried extracts.

Potential Dangers

No known drug interactions, side effects, or contraindications.

LICORICE ROOT

Glycyrrhiza glabra

Nearly everyone knows the sweet taste of licorice (even if the flavor in candies usually comes from another herb, anise). True licorice is used in cough medicines, with the medicinal value coming from the sweet-tasting root. Native to Europe, with spiky, blue flowers, licorice is a member of the pea family, and is a perennial herb.

Potential Health Benefits

The midnight-black extract of the root is effective for curing inflammation of the upper respiratory tract, according to the commission, which also concludes that the glycyrrhizic acid in licorice helps to heal gastric and duodenal ulcers. However, licorice juice, also used medicinally, wasn't endorsed by Commission E.

Scientific Evidence

The glycyrrhizic acid in licorice root helps to heal ulcers and loosens mucous, which enhances licorice's value in treating bronchitis and coughs. According to a 1992 study published in *Microbiology and Immunology*, licorice stimulates the production of interferon, which in turn fights viruses. In studies published in the *Lancet*, the *British Medical Journal*, and the *Journal of the American Medical Association*, licorice has performed well in tests measuring its effectiveness against the herpes simplex virus.

How to Use the Herb

Licorice is taken internally. Commission E's recommendations: average daily doses of 5–15 grams of powdered root, equivalent to

200–600 milligrams of glycrrhizin. With liquid extracts, 0.5–1.0 gram for inflammation of the upper respiratory tract and 1.5–3.0 grams per day for gastric/duodenal ulcers.

Consumer Products Available

Teas, as well as dried, powdered root, are sold in health food stores and cough medicines are available in drugstores.

Potential Dangers

Licorice is useful but tricky. It shouldn't be used medically by persons with liver disorders or severe kidney insufficiency or by pregnant or nursing women. Avoid licorice if you have a history of heart problems or stroke; it can cause potassium loss and water retention, elevating blood pressure. Don't use for more than four to six weeks without medical supervision. According to American nutritionist Ed Blonz, licorice root poses "potential interactions with digitalis drugs, thiazide or loop diuretics: corticosteroids, and aspirin or other anti-inflammatory drugs."

Marshmallow

Althaea officinalis

Forget the spongy white concoctions we toast over campfires and call marshmallows; there's no marshmallow in them, just sugar and starch. The real marshmallow herb was enjoyed for centuries as a sweet treat, and was also known as sweetweed. It was used as medicine, as well, and still is. Both the leaf and the root of marshmallow, a native of central Asia found near marshes and sporting large, pink flowers, are used medicinally.

Potential Health Benefits

The dried leaf of marshmallow is employed to coat an irritated, inflamed throat and treat dry cough. The root has the same uses as the leaf, and is additionally used to soothe an upset stomach.

Scientific Evidence

The mucilage in preparations made from marshmallow root and leaf coat the mouth, throat, and stomach by swelling and forming a gel when combined with water. American health writer Michael Castleman reports that marshmallow strengthened white blood cells against disease-producing microbes in one experiment. In animal tests, he adds, the root reduced blood sugar levels, suggesting that marshmallow could prove beneficial to diabetics.

How to Use the Herb

Marshmallow is taken internally. The doses for crushed, dried leaf is 5 grams daily. For crushed marshmallow root, the dose is 6 grams daily. For syrup, 10 grams per dose for treating coughs.

Consumer Products Available

Marshmallow preparations (not the sweet snacks) are available in health food stores and herb shops in the form of dried leaves, syrup, and tincture.

Potential Dangers

Diabetics should check the sugar content of the syrup. Commission E warned that marshmallow root could delay absorption of other drugs. If you are using marshmallow root, be sure to tell your health care provider.

MILK THISTLE FRUIT

Silybum marianum

Milky white veins in the leaves account for the name of this relative of the artichoke. Native to Europe, this prickly plant can reach heights of six feet and has gone wild in North America, where it's considered an invasive weed. A very useful weed, though—its ripe fruit is a powerful medicine.

Potential Health Benefits

Milk thistle fruit can calm a dyspeptic stomach. In refined formulations, it's credited by Commission E and other medical authorities with shielding the liver against invasive toxins such as alcohol and industrial pollutants and even generating new liver cells. This is a good thing; the liver is the body's chief detoxifier. Hepatitis, cirrhosis, and inflammatory liver disease are all treated with milk thistle.

Scientific Evidence

More than most any herb, milk thistle, which has been widely tested, has scientific bonafides. Its medicinal value is traced to a group of flavonoid compounds collectively known as silymarin. Silymarin toughens the membranes of liver cells against invasive toxins, and steps up the body's production of beneficial enzymes. A 1989 study published in the *Journal of Hepatology* concluded that milk thistle can be useful in treating people with cirrhosis or hepatitis. An Italian study found that milk thistle reduced damage to the liver brought on by chronic use of prescription drugs, while Swedish doctors have successfully used milk thistle as an antidote for mushroom poisoning.

How to Use the Herb

Because milk thistle's silymarin compounds are not very water-soluble, teas aren't highly recommended. Daily dosage is 12–15 grams of the powdered herb in formulations, equivalent to 200–400 milligrams of silymarin. The best way to take milk thistle is in tablets or capsules; the supplements should be standardized to 70 percent silymarin when using milk thistle for supporting treatment in chronic hepatic cirrhosis or inflammatory liver disease, according to Commission E. As always, read the product labels.

Consumer Products Available

Health food stores sell capsules and tablets of dried, powdered milk thistle fruit and teas.

Potential Dangers

Milk thistle can have a mild laxative effect. There are no other known side effects, contraindications, or drug interactions.

When buying milk thistle supplements, you'll want to make sure the label specifies that the product contains silymarin, the active ingredient, standardized to 80 percent. GNC Herbal Plus Standardized Milk Thistle Capsules contain the desired 80 percent silymarin, according to the label, and the 200 milligram capsules contain a convenient amount. If you follow manufacturers' instructions and take 1–2 capsules 3 times a day, however, you could get up to three times Commission E's recommended amount. Future Biotics Silymarin Plus Tablets contain six additional active ingredients; again, more may not be better. In any case, the efficacy of many ambitious milk thistle combinations on the North American market hasn't been proven.

MINT OIL

Mentha x piperita

The cooling, refreshing action of mint is well-known, whether it's found in flavored chewing gum, menthol-spiked cigarettes, or candy after-dinner "mints"—which in ancient times were sprigs of actual, fresh mint. The most popular mints are spearmint and its more assertive cousin, peppermint, a natural hybrid of spearmint first recognized in England in 1696. Most herbalists favor peppermint for medicinal purposes; indeed, peppermint is the "mint oil" endorsed by Commission E.

Potential Health Benefits

Peppermint oil is recommended for flatulence, gallbladder disorders, and clearing up inflammation of the upper respiratory tract. It's also approved for external use, to soothe diffuse muscle pain. The active ingredient, menthol, is included in mainstream cold remedies such as Vicks Cough Drops and Mentholatum Cream. Menthol isn't found in spearmint.

Scientific Evidence

Mint oil is obtained by steam distillation of fresh, flowering herb, yielding liquid with at least 42 percent menthol. The commission reports that medicinal amounts of menthol-rich oil stimulates bile flow, has cooling action, relieves gas, and exhibits antibacterial qualities. Studies published in the *American Journal of Gastroenterology* in 1997 and 1998 found enteric-coated peppermint oil capsules effective at treating irritable bowel syndrome. In a 1996 German study, 54 IBS patients given a capsule with 90 milligrams of peppermint oil extract combined with 50 milligrams of caraway oil far outpaced a placebo group in reporting beneficial results. In 1994, researchers found peppermint and eucalyptus oil as effective as aspirin at relieving tension headache when the mixed oil was spread on the skin.

How to Use the Herb

Mint teas are calming and delicious, although Commission E endorsed the oil, not the teas, for medicinal use. Mint oil can be consumed in water, at average daily doses of 3–6 drops; or you can put 3–4 drops in hot water for inhalation. For external use, try several drops of mint oil or commercial semisolid preparations, rubbed on the skin.

Consumer Products Available

Health food stores, herb shops, and supermarkets stock fresh mint and mint teas. Drugstores offer mainstream remedies with peppermint, such as Ben-Gay and Noxema skin cream. Health food stores also sell oil and extracts.

Potential Dangers

Upset stomach may occur for a few folks who take high doses rich in essential oil. More seriously, people with obstruction of the bile ducts, inflamed gallbladder, or severe liver damage shouldn't use mint oil. Keep preparations with mint oil away from the faces of infants and young children, due to their strong, concentrated quality. There are no known drug interactions.

MISTLETOE HERB

Viscum album

The Christmas kissing plant has a long but controversial history in medicine, owing to its potential toxicity. In Europe, the plant's leaves and flowers are used medically, and mistletoe tea is entrenched in folk medicine. Commission E studied European mistletoe, which is similar to the North American variety. Both are parasitic shrubs that grow in the branches of trees. Mistletoe is gathered from the wild.

Potential Health Benefits

Commission E considers mistletoe a serious drug, to be used carefully and under medical supervision. Mistletoe preparations are injected to treat degenerative inflammation of the joint: that is, rheumatoid arthritis. In Germany, mistletoe extract is also used as an anticancer drug (a use that hasn't been approved in the U.S.), and to lower blood pressure.

Scientific Evidence

Commission E doesn't cite scientific studies in its approval of mistletoe. Instead, its endorsement is drawn from the experience using mistletoe as part of German medical practice.

How to Use the Herb

Commission E approves fresh plant or cut and powdered herb for injections, but doesn't specify dose levels, perhaps to discourage consumers from using the drug on their own. American herbal writer Varro E. Tyler, Ph.D., flatly declares that "Mistletoe as a home remedy or as a beverage should definitely be avoided."

Consumer Products Available

Despite some herbalists' warnings, mistletoe teas and powdered herb can be found in health food stores and herb shops. The wreathed branches, complete with white berries, are widely sold at Christmas, but don't eat the berries!

Potential Dangers

The berries are considered toxic, especially for small children, by most authorities. Commission E doesn't comment on the berries, specifically, but does recommend caution when using mistletoe preparations. The commission notes that injections can cause swelling. Side effects can include "chills, high fever, headaches, angina, orthostatic circulatory disturbances and allergic reactions." Pregnant women shouldn't use mistletoe, and neither should people with "chronic-progressive infections," such as tuberculosis or AIDS.

MOTHERWORT HERB

Leonurus cardiaca

Motherwort is an Old World member of the mint family that has migrated to the New World. It has small leaves and prickly red and purple flowers. It has a faintly bitter taste. Its other name, heartwort, signals its medicinal value.

Potential Health Benefits

The aboveground parts of motherwort, gathered during flowering season, then dried and ground, are approved for calming heart palpitations and an overactive thyroid gland.

Scientific Evidence

The plant contains alkaloids and bitter principles, according to Commission E. Just how it works is uncertain to authorities. In this regard, motherwort is something of a mystery herb, not withstanding its long history of medicinal use in the Western world. In China, researchers found that motherwort reduced blood-clotting implicated in heart attacks, according to a 1983 report in the *Journal of Traditional Chinese Medicine*. Comprehensive Western studies using human test subjects evidently remain to be done.

How to Use the Herb

Ground, dried motherwort is taken internally in infusions. The average daily dosage is 4.5 grams, according to Commission E, which cites only doses of dried herb. *The PDR Family Guide to Natural Medicines & Healing Therapies* additionally recommends 5 drops of extract or tincture, or 1 tablet per day for an unspecified term.

Consumer Products Available

Health food stores sell motherwort in fluid extracts, tinctures, and tablets.

Potential Dangers

There are no known side effects, contraindications, or drug interactions from medicinal doses.

MULLEIN FLOWER

Verbascum densiflorum

A tall plant with velvety leaves and bright yellow flowers, mullein is also known as velvet plant and felt wort. It's well-known in both the Old World and the New as a medicinal plant, with the leaves, flowers, and roots being used. Commission E has endorsed the flower and its preparations.

Potential Health Benefits

The dried petals of mullein are used as an expectorant; many herbalists use it to treat coughs.

Scientific Evidence

The herb contains saponins and astringent tannins. It includes mucilage, a substance that coats the inside of the throat when it absorbs water and soothes irritated tissue. Extracts from mullein flowers have shown intriguing powers in clinical studies. In a 1991 European study, mullein extract was judged to have antiviral action against influenzas A and B as well as the herpes simplex virus —pointing to possible future uses of this herb.

How to Use the Herb

Mullein flowers, dried and ground, are taken at daily dosages of 3–4 grams. A tea can be made, as well, by pouring boiling water over 1.5–2.0 grams and steeping for 10 minutes.

Consumer Products Available

Dried flowers and teas are available in health food stores.

Potential Dangers

There are no known side effects, contraindications, or drug inter-actions.

ONION

Allium cepa

Onions are so common in cookery that they can be overlooked in the pharmacy. But onion, like its close herbal relative, garlic, can do more than flavor soups and stews and bring tears to your eyes.

Potential Health Benefits

Onion is okayed to restore appetite and for the prevention of arteriosclerosis. Onion can thin the blood and prevent clotting, helping to lower blood pressure. Onions are high in helpful fiber and low in calories.

Scientific Evidence

The sulfur compound in onions is credited for the plant's beneficial effects on the blood. Onion also has antibacterial qualities. Onions are exceptionally good sources of a helpful bioflavonoid called quercetin. In Asia, researchers theorize that quercetin helps inhibit cataracts associated with diabetes. American herbalist James A. Duke, Ph.D., alludes to a scientific study that found onions and garlic extracts to be useful against chronic asthma. Duke also writes that the quercetin in onions is helpful for "inhibiting tumors, thinning the blood, lowering blood pressure, and relieving asthma and pain." Duke endorses onions themselves over quercetin supplements sold in health food stores to combat hay fever and asthma, on the grounds that whole foods are the best medicine.

How to Use the Herb

Fresh, dried, as juice, or as syrup. The average daily dose is 50 grams of fresh onions or 20 grams of dried onions, according to Commission E. *The PDR Family Guide to Natural Medicines & Healing Therapies*, for its part, recommends 4–5 teaspoonfuls daily of tincture or 4–5 tablespoonfuls daily of onion syrup.

Consumer Products Available

Fresh onions are, of course, available everywhere. Health food stores and supermarkets also sell dried onion flakes, though syrup is harder to find; try the pharmacy.

Potential Dangers

You can get an upset stomach from eating lots of onions, and, of course, fierce breath. Other than that, there are no known side effects, contraindications, or drug interactions.

ORANGE PEEL

Citrus sinensis

Yes, the peel of the popular fruit can be, and is, used as medicine. Here's how:

Potential Health Benefits

Orange peel is used to stimulate the appetite. The fresh or dried outer peel of ripe oranges is used, after the white inner pulp is separated out.

Scientific Evidence

Commission E offers scant data about what makes orange peel effective, but gives its endorsement. Both bitter principles and aromatic essential oil are found in the peel.

How to Use the Herb

The daily dosage is 10–15 grams of fresh or dried peel, taken in tea.

Consumer Products Available

Health food stores and supermarkets are full to bursting with fresh oranges, and sell teas in which orange peel is an ingredient.

Potential Dangers

There are no known contraindications or drug interactions. No side effects are noted either, although the essential oil could conceivably cause gastric distress.

PAPRIKA
(RED PEPPER OR CAYENNE)

Capsicum annuum

Some like it hot—many do, in fact. That is why the numerous varieties of red-hot chile peppers are so popular as spices in cookery, as decorative objects in the pantry, even as the active ingredients in pepper sprays for self-defense. Commission E studied one type of red pepper, called paprika in German and French, also often called cayenne. (Actually, only pepper from the town of Cayenne, in French Guiana, is true cayenne.) Red peppers, native to South America, are grown in many parts of the world. Medicinal preparations are made from the dried fruits of various related species.

Potential Health Benefits

Commission E endorses paprika for external use, mainly to treat muscle pain in the shoulders, arms, and back. Many herbalists also use it internally to stimulate the appetite. Taken orally, red pepper opens up clogged mucous membranes and promotes perspiration, making it useful for treating colds and flu. Samuel Thomson (1769–1843), a popular 19th-century American health evangelist, used cayenne as a key ingredient in his Number 2 remedy, which was intended to effect cures by inducing sweating and purging.

Scientific Evidence

The active ingredient in paprika is capsaicin, which acts as a pain desensitizer. It knocks out what researchers have dubbed Substance P, a neurotransmitter compound that carries perception of pain to the spinal cord through the peripheral nerves. A 1985 Canadian study endorsed the value of capsaicin as a counterirritant—a substance that induces minor, local pain when applied to the skin, so that the body temporarily focuses on that instead of a greater pain elsewhere. A 1989 study published in the journal *Environmental Nutrition* showed that people suffering from cluster headaches who applied a capsaicin preparation inside and outside their noses noticed relief from pain within five days. All told, 75 percent of the test subjects reported at least some headache relief, pointing to another possible medicinal use of red pepper.

How to Use the Herb

Commission E recommends for external use: creams with 0.02–0.05 percent capsaicinoids, used 4 to 5 times per day; liquid preparations with 0.005–0.01 percent capsaicinoids; poultices containing 10–40 grams of capsaicinoids per square centimeter. If you're using creams externally, don't use them for more than 2 days, and wait 14 days before using them again on the same part of the body. Health writer Michael Castleman recommends ¼–½ teaspoonful of dried red pepper per cup of boiling water for an infusion, taken after meals.

Consumer Products Available

Drugstores sell over-the-counter creams Zostrix and Axsain, both with capsaicin as an ingredient, for chronic pain; both have USFDA approval. Fresh and dried red peppers are available in supermarkets. Health food stores and supermarkets carry red pepper extracts and capsules, which should be taken with food.

Potential Dangers

Red pepper is powerful medicine. Long-term external use can cause nerve damage. If you handle red peppers, be very careful not to rub your eyes or other sensitive areas and consider using rubber gloves. Use vinegar (not water) to wash bare hands after handling red peppers. Don't use capsaicin creams on wounds or infections. If you use red pepper internally, err on the side of caution until you determine the dose that's right for you. Red pepper has no known drug interactions.

PARSLEY

Petroselinum crispum

This common garnish for the dinner plate is a native of the Mediterranean region and a biennial herb. Commission E evaluated the root and above-ground body of the plant for medicinal qualities.

Potential Health Benefits

The commission recommends using parsley for flushing out the urinary tract and for the prevention and treatment of kidney stones. Folklore additionally credits parsley with increasing menstrual flow and inducing abortion. In Europe, parsley tea is favored for its diuretic effect, and as a means of dealing with high blood pressure —a use not specifically endorsed by the commission. The high chlorophyll content in parsley accounts for its value as a breath freshener.

Scientific Evidence

The active chemicals in parsley include apiol and myristicin, which account for its diuretic effect and have mild laxative power. In his book *Tyler's Honest Herbal*, plant pharmacologist Varro E. Tyler, Ph.D., comments: "Both apiol and myristicin are uterine stimulants, accounting for the use of parsley volatile oil as an emmenagogue [promoting menstruation] and for its misuse as an abortifacient [promoting abortion]." A 1979 study in the *American Journal of Chinese Medicine* suggests that parsley may help lower blood pressure, although this use hasn't been widely studied.

How to Use the Herb

Commission E specifies 6 grams of dried root or herb, taken with plenty of water. Other sources offer additional ways of using parsley medicinally. *The PDR Family Guide to Natural Medicines & Healing Therapies* recommends parsley tea 2 to 3 times per day, using tea bags of crushed leaf and root. Health writer Michael Castleman suggests ½–1 teaspoonfuls of tincture as many as 3 times per day for use as a laxative and diuretic.

Consumer Products Available

Fresh and dried parsley is widely available in health food stores and supermarkets. Health food stores also sell parsley tinctures. Parsley is frequently included in garlic supplements to sweeten the breath.

Potential Dangers

Essential oil made from parsley seeds, which haven't been as well-tested as the root and plant, is powerful stuff and shouldn't be used by itself. Pregnant women shouldn't use medicinal amounts of parsley, nor should anyone with swelling caused by heart or kidney disease. Skin rashes in sensitive individuals can occur. There are no known drug interactions.

PEPPERMINT
Mencha piperita

While peppermint, combined with spearmint, is the main source of the mint oil approved by Commission E, the commission thought so highly of peppermint, it gave the herb two more monographs: one for the leaf and one for the oil. We have combined them into one entry on peppermint, which is a hybrid derived from spearmint and considered both more powerful and more versatile than spearmint.

Potential Health Benefits

Commission E commends peppermint leaf for its ability to quiet spasms of the gastrointestinal tract, gallbladder, and bile ducts. The commission endorses the essential oil—which is steam-distilled from dried peppermint leaf—for all those treatments, plus some others. They include inflammations of the respiratory tract and inflammation of the mouth. For external use, Commission E endorses peppermint oil for effective relief of muscle pain and neuralgia (nerve inflammation).

Scientific Evidence

The herb contains at least 1.2 percent essential oil, whose main active ingredient is menthol. According to Varro E. Tyler, Ph.D., in his book *Tyler's Honest Herbal*, "American peppermint oil contains from 50 to 78 percent of free menthol and another 5 to 20 percent of various combined forms of [esters] of menthol. Those major components are also largely responsible for the peppermint's ability to stimulate bile flow and promote digestion." A German study in 1996 found a mixture of 90 milligrams of peppermint oil and 50 milligrams of caraway, taken in coated capsules, effective in treating upset stomach. A 1994 study published in the journal *Cephalalgia* found a combination of peppermint oil and eucalyptus oil as effective as aspirin for treating headaches when the mixed oils were rubbed on the skin. Commission E doesn't cite this use of peppermint oil, alone or in combination.

How to Use the Herb

The recommended internal dose of peppermint leaf is 3–6 grams. To make tea, pour ½ cup of hot water over 1 teaspoonful of leaves, steep for 10 minutes, and strain; drink up to 3 cups per day. For internal use of potent concentrated oil, the average daily dose is 6–12 drops in water; for inhalation, 3–4 drops in hot water; for irritable bowel syndrome, the average single dose is 0.6 milliliters in coated tablets.

For external use of the oil, look for 5–20 percent essential oil in creams and ointments, 1–5 percent in nasal ointments.

Consumer Products Available

Health food stores and supermarkets sell fresh and dried leaf. Health food stores also sell tinctures, tablets, ointments, and dry extracts of peppermint oil.

Potential Dangers

People with gallstones should consult a physician before using peppermint leaves. Obstructed bile ducts, severe liver damage, and gallbladder infection rule out use of the powerful essential oil. Peppermint oil should be kept away from the faces of small children and not used externally on infants or small children. There are no known drug interactions.

PLANTAIN

Plantago lanceolasta

The plantain approved by Commission E is often regarded as a mere weed. Introduced to North America from Europe, it has broad, ribbed leaves and draws its name from the Latin word *plantago*, which means "foot," because its leaves are shaped somewhat like a human foot. (This plant isn't the plantain palm that produces the banana-like fruit popular in Latin American cuisine; that's *Musa paradisiaca*.)

Potential Health Benefits

Plantain herb is used to cure inflammation of the upper respiratory tract, treat infections of the mouth, and loosen mucous in persons with colds or flu. The fresh or dried above-ground parts of the plant are used medicinally; they're harvested at flowering time.

Scientific Evidence

Commission E offers little hard data on plantain, which seems to be little-known among other herbal researchers. Based on years of use in German pharmacies (as differentiated from controlled clinical studies), the commission ascribes antibacterial qualities to the plant, as well as astringent action.

How to Use the Herb

Plantain herb is used both internally and externally in dried form. Internally, the average daily dosage is 3–6 grams of the dried herb. Externally, it can be mixed with water and swabbed on inflamed skin.

Consumer Products Available

Plantain isn't one of the more widely known or widely distributed herbs, but it can be useful. Health food stores and herb shops are the most likely sources.

Potential Dangers

There are no known side effects, contraindications, or drug interactions.

POLLEN

Pollen

Pollen is the yellow powdery stuff on the stamens of flowers; it's the plant's male sex cells. Commission E ascribes medicinal qualities to pollen, collected from what the commission generically terms "various flowering plants." This, please note, isn't necessarily bee pollen (propolis), often sold in health food stores as a near-panacea and said to have been collected by bees from poplar and conifer trees—a hard-to-verify claim. Propolis, a brown, resinous material, wasn't evaluated by the commission.

Potential Health Benefits

Although pollen, as male sex cells, sounds like it would be more exciting for plants than people, Commission E considers it a roborant —a quaint term meaning a strengthening agent or tonic. Pollen, the commission concludes, is useful for reversing "feebleness and loss of appetite."

Scientific Evidence

Commission E doesn't endorse pollen for many of the wide range of uses that herbal enthusiasts claim it's good for. Such uses allegedly include: slowing the aging process, treating anemia, and mitigating colitis. In any case, pollen is highly variable; its composition depends on where and when it's collected. Controlled clinical studies of pollen seem to be scarce, but Germans have long used it to stimulate appetite, and Commission E aligns itself with this empirical evidence.

How to Use the Herb

The average daily dose is 30–40 grams of pollen, taken with water, to stimulate the appetite and act as a pick-me-up.

Consumer Products Available

Pollen is available in health food stores, in tablets and capsules.

Potential Dangers

Don't use commercial pollen preparations if you're allergic to raw pollen. Rarely, pollen can cause gastric distress. There are no known drug interactions.

PRIMROSE

Primula vertis and Primula elatior

The primrose path is lined with white, red, and yellow flowers, the blooms on an early-flowering plant also known as cowslip, butter rose, and fairy cap. Commission E issued separate monographs on the flower and root, the parts of the primrose that are used medicinally. Since most of that information overlaps, we have melded the two monographs into one. (Note: The evening primrose, *Oenothera biennis*, wasn't reviewed.) This native of central Europe grows up to eight inches high.

Potential Health Benefits

Primrose flower and root are used for the same maladies: clearing up inflammation of the respiratory tract. Commission E endorses that single use; it doesn't endorse claims by primrose enthusiasts that the plant cures headaches, strengthens the heart, or helps treat asthma and gout.

Scientific Evidence

Citing the empirical use of primrose in Germany, the commission concludes that both common forms of primrose are expectorants with secretolytic abilities: that is, they slow secretions in the body, helping to subdue bronchitis and cough. The commission also notes that saponins are prominent ingredients of primrose. Saponins, taken orally, act as respiratory irritants, which is why traditional herbalists prescribe saponin-containing mixtures as expectorants, according to Steven B. Karch, M.D., author of *The Consumer's Guide to Herbal Medicine.*

How to Use the Herb

The daily dosage for dried primrose flower is 2–4 grams of the plant and 2.5–7.5 grams of tincture. For dried root, the daily dose is 0.5–1.5 grams, or 1.5–3.0 grams of the tincture, according to Commission E. Primrose can also be taken as tea. *The PDR Family Guide to Natural Medicines & Healing Therapies* recommends primrose flower tea of 2–4 grams steeped in hot water for 10 minutes, then taken throughout the day. For root tea, 0.2–0.5 grams of fine-cut powder steeped in cold water for 5 minutes and taken every 2 to 3 hours.

Consumer Products Available

Health food stores sell primrose in a variety of forms: dried flowers, extracts, and tinctures. It's often a prime ingredient in cough syrups and mixed herbal teas.

Potential Dangers

Some people are allergic to primrose, and gastric discomfort and nausea can result from both flowers and roots. There are no known drug interactions.

PSYLLIUM SEED, BLACK

Plantago indica

Commission E actually issues three evaluations of psyllium, an herbal laxative that's the main ingredient in Metamucil, Pro-lax, and other mainstream products. We follow the commission's lead with a summary of black psyllium seed; for blonde psyllium seed and blonde seed husk, which are similar, we have written a second, separate profile. Psyllium is an annual that produces brown, seed-bearing pods. The plant is also sometimes called plantain, but shouldn't be confused with the plantain herb covered elsewhere in this book, nor with the banana-like palm also known as plantain.

Potential Health Benefits

The dried, ripe black seeds from psyllium are used to clear up chronic constipation and irritable bowel syndrome. Like the blonde seeds, black seed has recently been shown to have valuable cholesterol-lowering properties.

Scientific Evidence

The mucilage in psyllium seeds combines with water in the intestines. The water-logged bulk speeds stools on their way, helping to end constipation. Psyllium can help control diarrhea, too, since the added water and mucilage add bulk to stools. Psyllium's cholesterol-fighting qualities have been demonstrated in controlled studies. In a 1988 study published in the *Archives of Internal Medicine*, 3 teaspoonfuls of psyllium daily for 8 weeks lowered the blood cholesterol levels of human test subjects. A 1989 study published in the *Journal of the American Medical Association* showed that psyllium reduced cholesterol in people taking it for 12 weeks by an average of 5 percent, lowering the risk of heart attack.

How to Use the Herb

The ground seeds are used in 10–30 gram dosages. Take with plenty of water; 1–2 glasses per dose is standard. Wait 30–60 minutes to take psyllium if you're taking other medications; otherwise, psyllium may delay the absorption of these medicines.

Consumer Products Available

Health food stores and drugstores stock psyllium powder, pills, and capsules.

Potential Dangers

Narrowing of the esophagus or the gastrointestinal tract precludes the use of psyllium. Diabetics should consult their physician before taking psyllium.

PSYLLIUM SEED, BLONDE

Plantago isphagula

Commission E and other herbal researchers don't champion blonde or black seed psyllium over the other. However, the commission notes that a wider range of conditions can be treated with blonde seed and its husk. Like black seed, blonde psyllium is a natural source of fiber.

Potential Health Benefits

Same as black psyllium seed. Plus, Commission E finds additional uses for blonde seed husk, declaring it to be helpful for patients who have had anal/rectal surgery, for pregnancy-induced constipation, and as a secondary treatment for various kinds of diarrhea.

Scientific Evidence

The commission doesn't cite additional reasons for using blonde seed and its husk instead of the black seed, nor do other herbal writers we surveyed.

How to Use the Herb

The dosage is higher than with black seed. For blonde seed, take 12–40 grams per day with plenty of water. For blonde seed husk, the range of doses is quite wide: 4–20 grams per day, again with plenty of water.

Consumer Products Available

Same as with black seed.

Potential Dangers

If diarrhea lasts more than 3–4 days, consult a physician. The commission also cautions diabetics using blonde seed or blonde seed husks that "There may need to be a reduction in the insulin usage in diabetics that are insulin-dependent." If gas or bloating results from using psyllium, try another laxative such as flaxseed oil.

PUMPKIN SEED

Cucurbita papo

The Halloween gourd—big, holiday-orange, filled with hundreds of oblong seeds—is familiar to virtually everyone in North America, where pumpkin is a native plant. Today, pumpkins are grown in many places around the world, including the tropics. The seeds are the medicinal part.

Potential Health Benefits

Pumpkin seed is widely used to treat urinary problems, especially in men affected by benign prostate hypertrophy (BPH), a non-cancerous enlargement of the prostate gland associated with aging. In traditional Asian medicine, pumpkin seed is used to treat worms and diabetes, although scientists haven't confirmed pumpkin's value for such uses.

Scientific Evidence

Commission E says of pumpkin seed: "Due to the lack of suitable modeling, there are no pharmacological studies that substantiate the empirically found clinical activity." The seeds appear to have anti-inflammatory properties, although researchers aren't quite sure how or why. Elevated levels of the male hormone dihydrotestosterone (DHT) are associated with enlarged prostate glands. In *Dr. Duke's Essential Herbs*, James A. Duke, Ph.D., reports "In one study, BPH patients took 90 milligrams of isolated pumpkin sterols before undergoing surgery to remove their prostates. Tissue analyses later confirmed that the pumpkin users' glands contained less DHT."

How to Use the Herb

Commission E recommends using coarsely ground seed at an average daily dose of 10 grams, taken with water, morning and evening.

Consumer Products Available

Whole and ground pumpkin seeds are available in health food stores. The whole seeds are, of course, available in pumpkins; toasted and lightly salted, they're a tasty snack.

Potential Dangers

There are no known side effects, contraindications, or drug interactions. Be advised, though, that pumpkin seeds treat only the symptoms of BPH and inflamed urinary tracts; they don't cure the underlying diseases.

RADISH

Raphanus sativus

The radish is a familiar feature of the modern supermarket and grocery store, where it's valued for its bright red color, pleasantly peppery taste, and crunchy texture. Radishes also have medicinal value, concentrated in the roots.

Potential Health Benefits

Radish root is used to treat spasms in the bile ducts as well as catarrhs of the upper respiratory tract. In medicine, it isn't the pulp that's used directly, but pressed juice from the root.

Scientific Evidence

Radish root contains tangy mustard oil glycosides and essential oil, which stimulates digestive juices, kills microbes, and stimulates the bowels.

How to Use the Herb

Fresh, whole radishes are widely available. Fresh juice can be obtained from grated or pressed radishes. Commission E prescribes 50–100 milliliters of juice daily, taken several times during the day. To treat the symptoms of whooping cough, *The PDR Family Guide to Natural Medicines & Healing Therapies* recommends grating a radish into honey and allowing it to settle for 10 hours before spooning it down.

Consumer Products Available

Radishes are widely sold in supermarkets and health food stores; the latter occasionally have radish juice, as well.

Potential Dangers

There are no known side effects, contraindications, or drug interactions.

RHUBARB ROOT

Rheum palmatum

Medicinal rhubarb isn't the same form of the plant used in pies; that's *rheum rhapositum*. As medicine, the *rheum palmatum* variety has a long history of use as a tonic and a laxative. Commission E endorses its use as a laxative. Growing up to ten feet tall, medical rhubarb, a plant native to the Volga River Valley of Russia, centers its active properties in the dried roots, stripped of stems and bark. (The stalks of garden rhubarb, which can grow about three feet high, are the parts used in cooking—be advised that the leaves are poisonous.)

Potential Health Benefits

Commission E reports that rhubarb promotes secretions in the bowel and stomach and stimulates propulsive contractions while increasing the water and electrolyte content of the stool. All this makes it an effective laxative.

Scientific Evidence

Commission E reports that "Systematic studies pertaining to the genotoxicity of rhubarb preparations are not available." In addition, the commission observes that "Experiments pertaining to the genotoxicity of rhubarb and its preparations are not available. No data are available for carcinogenicity." The commission's recommendations are drawn from the empirical use of the plant in Germany. The laxative-inducing chemicals in rhubarb, anthraquinones, are also found in buckhorn.

How to Use the Herb

The average daily dosage is 20–30 milligrams, or "the smallest dosage necessary to maintain a soft stool." Additionally, in *The Healing Herbs*, Michael Castleman recommends 1 cup of rhubarb tea per day to alleviate constipation.

Consumer Products Available

Health food stores sell rhubarb as powdered extracts for teas, and as a tincture.

Potential Dangers

Taking rhubarb preparations for more than two weeks can make you dependent on them, so do limit use. Pregnant and lactating women shouldn't use rhubarb. Rhubarb can cause a potassium deficiency, which can contribute to heart disorders and muscular weakness and can strengthen the action of heart medications such as digitalis. People with appendicitis, intestinal blockage, or Crohn's disease shouldn't use rhubarb. As with any laxative, rhubarb should be used only after making dietary changes: for example, after adding more bulk and fiber has been tried first. Rhubarb is contraindicated for children.

ROSE FLOWER

Rosa centifolia

"A rose is a rose is a rose," except when it's a medicine. Native to Asia, perhaps to Iran, roses eventually entered the pharmacopeia in Europe. Hippocrates, the father of Western medicine, prescribed rose flowers and oil for uterine disease, and the 10th-century Arab physician Avicenna used rose water as a medicine.

In our era, rose hips—the cherry-sized fruit of the rose—are prized as natural sources of vitamin C. Commission E studied rose petals, dried and collected prior to fully unfolding. Interestingly, Commission E concluded that rose hip preparations made from *Rosa canina*, a particular kind of rose also known as dog rose, are ineffective, and placed rose hips on its list of unapproved herbs.

Potential Health Benefits

Commission E recommends rose flowers—chiefly in the form of teas and mouthwash—as treatments for "mild inflammations of the oral and pharyngeal mucosa": sore throat. In traditional Asian medicine, rose flowers have been used to reduce sweating and treat coughs, uses that the commission didn't address.

Scientific Evidence

Clinical studies of rose petals are few; Commission E drew its conclusions from the long history of the rose in German medicine. Not all herbal authorities agree with the commission's dismissal of rose hips. *The Canadian Medical Association Journal* cites several studies in the 1970s using large doses of rose hip–derived vitamin C (up to 2,000 milligrams per day) to lessen the severity and duration of colds; however, if rose hips were the sole source of vitamin

C, one would have to sip rose hip tea practically nonstop to get enough vitamin C just from the plant source. As for rose petals, their usefulness comes mainly from tannins, which give the flowers astringent properties.

How to Use the Herb

Commission E recommends 1–2 grams of dried rose petal preparations per cup, taken as tea, several times per day. There are no recommendations for unapproved rose hips.

Consumer Products Available

Teas made from rose petals are available in health food stores and supermarkets. Vitamin C supplements with rose hips are commonplace in health food stores, supermarkets, and pharmacies. However, observes health writer Michael Castleman in his book *The Healing Herbs*, "the drying process destroys from 45 to 90 percent" of the vitamin C in rose hips, and "infusions extract only about 40 percent of what's left." Rose hips are sometimes added to laboratory-synthesized ascorbic acid, the source of most vitamin C supplements, but rose hips mainly raise the price of the products.

Potential Dangers

Roses appear to be as benign as they are beautiful. There are no known interactions with other drugs, or adverse side effects from rose flowers (or rose hips, for that matter).

ROSEMARY LEAF
Rosmarinus officinalis

This perennial herb with pretty blue flowers is native to the Mediterranean region. A member of the mint family, it's associated in herbal lore with memory. Commission E didn't credit rosemary with having any effect on memory, but did find preparations made from rosemary leaves to be effective for upset stomach when taken internally, and for easing circulatory complaints when used externally.

Potential Health Benefits

Like many herbs, rosemary has been credited with working medical wonders. In the Middle Ages, for example, people used rosemary oil in vain hopes of warding off the Black Death. However, the aromatic essential oil of rosemary, which is drawn from the leaves, does have medicinal value. In addition to the uses cited above, Commission E endorses rosemary oil, used externally, as a supportive therapy for rheumatism.

Scientific Evidence

Studies credit rosemary with strong antioxidant qualities; used in food preparation, this popular culinary herb helps slow the oxidizing effect that makes the fats in meat turn rancid. Commission E also declares that rosemary's essential oil, when added to a hot bath, can stimulate the circulation. Varro E. Tyler, Ph.D., writing in his book *Tyler's Honest Herbal*, attributes rosemary's physiological power to "its volatile oil, which occurs in the leaves in concentrations ranging from 1 to 2.5 percent."

How to Use the Herb

Commission E suggests a daily dosage of 4–6 grams of the herb, or 10–20 drops of essential oil, taken internally. (However, the American Botanical Council, an herb industry group, demurs, warning that "The essential oil dosage appears excessive and possibly unsafe. A more reasonable dosage for internal use would be 2 drops.") Alternately, American health writer Michael Castleman recommends taking ¼–½ teaspoonful of rosemary tincture up to 3 times per day "to settle the stomach or clear a stuffed nose." For external use, *The PDR Family Guide to Natural Medicines & Healing Therapies* recommends mixing 50 grams of essential oil into 1 liter of water as a bath additive.

Consumer Products Available

Fresh rosemary is available in supermarkets and health food stores. Health food stores also sell rosemary in powdered form as well as its essential oil.

Potential Dangers

Commission E finds no contraindications, side effects, or known interactions with other drugs. Some authorities advise pregnant women to avoid taking medicinal amounts of rosemary, as large dosages could possibly induce abortion.

SAGE

Salvia officinalis

Although sage is known in North America primarily as a flavoring for food, this perennial herb with gray-green aromatic leaves has a long history of medical use, especially in Europe. Sage is a member of the mint family and native of the Mediterranean region. Its scientific name, *Salvia*, comes from the Latin word for "to heal." At various times, sage was regarded as a virtual panacea. Commission E doesn't consider sage a panacea, but does verify its usefulness.

Potential Health Benefits

Commission E recommends sage leaf and preparations derived from sage leaves for treating inflammation of the mucous membranes of the nose and throat. Sage is also recommended for relieving dyspepsia and for drying up excessive perspiration. In Germany, a sage-based commercial preparation called Salvysat Burger is marketed as an antiperspirant.

Scientific Evidence

Sage contains tannins whose astringent properties help account for its use in Germany as treatment for sore throat, bleeding gums, and canker sores. In food preparation, sage, like rosemary, has antioxidants that help keep food from going rancid. Sage's powerful taste and smell come chiefly from camphor, one of its prime constituents. Commission E, without citing sources, credits sage with having antibiotic, antifungal, and antiviral powers. Sage may have antidiabetes qualities as well. A 1950 study published in Germany reported that blood sugar levels in test subjects were cut in half when they took liquid sage decoctions on an empty stomach. More study is needed to investigate this encouraging possibility.

How to Use the Herb

For internal use: Commission E's recommended daily dosage is 4–6 grams of dried sage, 2–6 drops of essential oil, 2.5–7.5 grams of tincture, or 1.5–3.0 grams of liquid extract. For external use: in a gargle or mouthwash Commission E recommends 2.5 grams of the herb; for an infusion, 2–3 drops of essential oil in 100 milliliters of water; for an alcoholic extract, 5 grams in 1 glass of water.

Consumer Products Available

Sage is available in health food stores and supermarkets in fresh and powdered form. Health food stores and pharmacies sell sage extracts, tinctures, and paste.

Potential Dangers

Commission E cautions that "After prolonged ingestion of alcohol extracts or of the pure essential oil, convulsions can occur." The commission also warns women that "The pure essential oil and alcoholic extracts should not be used internally during pregnancy." There are no known interactions with other drugs. *The PDR Family Guide to Natural Medicines & Healing Therapies* notes that overdoses could result from prolonged, regular usage of even prescribed medicinal amounts; in other words, sage is for short-term use.

SARSAPARILLA

Smilax officinalis

Sarsaparilla is a climbing vine native to Mexico, the Caribbean, and Brazil, with spiky, heart-shaped leaves. The root is a popular flavoring agent in carbonated soft drinks and is used in teas. Despite the long history of use, however, Commission E put the plant on its list of unapproved herbs. It's a controversial decision.

Potential Health Benefits

Sarsaparilla's champions say it can increase energy, act as a diuretic and laxative, and help bring down high blood pressure. In Germany, sarsaparilla has also been used to treat skin diseases such as psoriasis as well as kidney diseases, but Commission E concluded that "The claimed efficacy has not been documented" for treating these maladies.

Scientific Evidence

Sarsaparilla contains vitamins A and D and minerals such as sulfur and zinc, plus the steroid-like substances saporin, sarsapogenin, and smilagenin.

In a monograph published in 1990, Commission E concluded that the herb can cause gastric distress and temporary kidney dysfunction. Seven years later, one commission member disagreed, suggesting that the doses used had been too high. Most North American herbalists consider the plant safe.

How to Use the Herb

Beth Ann Petro Roybal and Gayle Skowronski, in their book *Sex Herbs*, suggest: "a common dose is one-fourth to one-half teaspoon of the tincture 1 to 3 times per day," to boost energy. They write that sarsparilla also "has the benefit of raising the sexual drive in both sexes. . . ." Follow instructions on product labels for tea.

Consumer Products Available

Teas, soft drinks, tinctures, and extracts are available in health food stores and markets.

Potential Dangers

Stomach upset, kidney dysfunction, and, Commission E warns, "increased or decreased action of [other] herbs taken simultaneously." Given the long and widespread use of this herb, we believe there's cause to debate the commission's low opinion of sarsaparilla.

SAW PALMETTO BERRY

Serenoa repens

The saw palmetto plant doesn't look like much: It's a short palm native to the southeastern United States, with spiked, fan-shaped leaves and small fruit about the size and color of dark olives. But the saw palmetto's fruit—more specifically, extracts of the berry—is valued as medicine. In Germany, it's a popular over-the-counter remedy.

Potential Health Benefits

Saw palmetto is used to relieve symptoms of benign prostatic hypertrophy (BPH), the noncancerous enlargement of the prostate gland. Saw palmetto doesn't shrink the gland, but it does ease annoying symptoms of BPH: frequent urination, weak urination, and sleep-destroying nighttime urination. Many men who use it report fewer side effects with saw palmetto than with synthetic drugs used to treat BPH.

Scientific Evidence

According to Commission E, "The drug contains fatty oils with phytosterols and polysaccharides." In tests, the extract of ripe, dried fruit appeared to relieve BPH symptoms by means of its antiandrogen and anti-inflammatory properties. A 1996 study of more than 1,000 men found saw palmetto as effective as the drug Proscar and lacking major side effects such as impotence and weak libido, according to the journal *Prostate*. European studies show that saw palmetto is especially effective in the early stages of BPH. A German study found that only 2 percent of male subjects dropped

Supplements of this useful herb should contain an extract standardized to 85 percent to 95 percent fatty acids and sterols, and should contain amounts of active ingredients close to Commission E's recommended amounts, to be convenient and medicinally useful. Drugstore.com Saw Palmetto Concentrate Softgels are set at 80 milligrams. Two capsules taken twice a day, as per the manufacturer's directions, would give the right amount of extract, although the product has 80 percent standardized fatty acids, just below recommended levels. GNC's Men's Prosta-Cern Herbal Supplement Tablets include lower levels of saw palmetto extract, which is standardized to 40–45 percent free fatty acids, plus a cluster of other ingredients such as vitamin E. Another product, One-a-Day Prostate Health, consists of softgels taken twice a day that provide 640 milligrams of saw palmetto berry extract, which is exactly Commission E's recommended amount. However, the product also contains pumpkin seed oil and zinc, also long associated with prostate health but not studied in combination by Commission E. As with other combinations, such products may prove useful, but there's less independent documentation of them than with single herbs, and combinations may be more complex than they need to be.

out of the trial because of side effects from saw palmetto, while some 80 percent reported an easing of their symptoms.

How to Use the Herb

Commission E used daily doses of 1–2 grams of the dried berry and 320 milligrams of berry extract; the latter is the standard dose in European clinical trials.

Consumer Products Available

Health food stores, drugstores, and supermarkets stock tinctures, extracts, and capsules containing saw palmetto. The herb is generally much cheaper than prescription drugs; figures published by James A. Duke, Ph.D., in his 1999 book *Dr. Duke's Essential Herbs*, estimated that a year's supply of saw palmetto supplements cost $180, compared to $600 for Proscar and $480 for Hytrin, another prescription drug.

Potential Dangers

In rare cases, enlarged breasts in men or stomach problems, although serious side effects aren't widespread and the commission found no known interactions with other drugs. Consult your doctor before supplementing with this herb, to make certain that an enlarged prostate is indeed benign.

ST. JOHN'S WORT

Hypericum perforatum

The feel-good best-seller of the modern herbal market, St. John's wort migrated from Europe and Asia with the colonists several centuries back. It now grows extensively in North America as a perennial shrub. It has oblong leaves and bright yellow, star-shaped flowers. St. John's wort was once harvested on and around St. John's Day (June 24). Wort (not wart) is an Old English word for plant, root, or herb.

Potential Health Benefits

The flowers of St. John's wort are considered the most medicinally active part of the plant, which has won renown as a treatment for mild depression. Taken internally, it improves mood and allays anxiety. In Germany, the plant far outsells Prozac. St. John's wort is also applied topically to treat burns, given that is has antibiotic qualities and is an anti-inflammatory agent. Additionally, Commission E recommends internal use to calm the stomach.

Scientific Evidence

The plant's most celebrated active ingredient is hypericin. Other as yet unknown chemicals may help give St. John's wort its power to fight depression, researchers believe, with the substance hyperflorin thought to be a likely candidate. According to a 1996 study in the British medical journal *Lancet*, a review of 23 tests of the herb, covering nearly 1,800 patients, found St. John's wort to be as effective as prescription drugs and with much milder side effects. In an article for *Prevention* magazine, Varro E. Tyler, dean emeritus of the Purdue University School of Pharmacy and Pharmacal

If you're buying St. John's wort supplements, you want to look for labels that specify 0.3 percent hypericin in the product, although other ingredients, especially hyperflorin, may be important, too. Also, pay attention to how much St. John's wort is actually in the product, and how convenient it is to use. For example, Nature's Answer St. John's Wort Alcohol-Free is a liquid taken in drops. The manufacturer helpfully specifies that the leaf, flower, and stem of the St. John's wort plant were used and recommends 14–28 drops, taken 3 times per day. You do the math. That's 42 to 84 drops of medicine per day. If that works for you, fine. Movana St. John's Wort Tablets, according to the manufacturer's label, contain a stabilized version of hyperflorin, the ingredient attracting the attention of researchers. Movana's label also specifies 0.3 hypericin, which is good, and identifies flowers and leaves as its sources of the herb, which is also good. More controversially, the company's label also states "Doses above 900 mg [milligrams] per day have not been shown [to have] any greater effectiveness." According to Commission E, they have. Then, too, there is the always-pertinent issue of price. When

I was finishing the research for this book, Dr. Art Ulene Herbal Formulas' Standardized St. John's Wort Capsules were retailing for $2.99, down from $4.99, for 30 capsules with 150 milligrams each. That's a low price, but the product also had a low dosage; you'd have to swallow anywhere from 7 to 18 capsules per day to be in Commission E's recommended daily range. Another product, Nature's Apothecary St. John's Wort Liquid Extract, uses organically grown herbs, according to the label. However, the label cites no documentation for the claim and lists no phone number or website. You may not need to use it, but it's always good to have contact information available should you have any questions, and in my view companies should routinely provide it.

Studies, cited German studies of 3,250 depressed patients, 80 percent of whom said they felt much less depressed after taking St. John's wort.

How to Use the Herb

Commission E recommends a daily dose of 2–4 grams for internal use. The standardized supplement dose in Germany for internal use contains 0.3 percent hypericin. The drug starts to work after about six weeks for patients with mild to moderate depression.

Consumer Products Available

St. John's wort is widely available in health food stores, supermarkets, and drugstores in tinctures, extracts, oils, and tablets. A 1998 laboratory test commissioned by the *Los Angeles Times* found that just three of ten supplement brands had the amount of St. John's wort claimed on product labels. Look for respected brands from companies with established track records.

Potential Dangers

Fair-skinned people may be photosensitive when taking St. John's wort. Although Commission E found no known interactions with other drugs, other observers' concern that St. John's wort could interact with other antidepressants prompted Ireland to require prescriptions for the herb. Alcohol intake should also be prudent in people using St. John's wort, as with any tranquilizer. In 2000, a U.S. study concluded that St. John's wort could weaken the effect of anti-HIV medicines, an important finding if verified by other scientists.

STAR ANISE SEED

Illicium verum

Still relatively little-known in the Western world, the star anise seed is the fruit of an evergreen tree native to China and used in traditional Asian medicine. The tree, which also grows in Vietnam, can reach 30 feet in height. The fruit (or seed) is eight-pointed, giving rise to its comparison to a star. Medicinal preparations are made by grinding fresh, ripe seeds.

Potential Health Benefits

Commission E endorses star anise as a treatment for inflammations of the respiratory tract and for relief from peptic discomforts. It loosens phlegm and helps soothe coughs and cure bronchitis, as well as calm spasms of the gastrointestinal tract. That makes it useful as a treatment for cramps, a long-time use of star anise in Asian medicine.

Scientific Evidence

Star anise appears to be scantily documented in Western scientific literature; indeed, Commission E produced a brief monograph on this useful herb, citing no sources.

How to Use the Herb

Fresh, ripe star anise should be ground just before use. Or, you can take 3 grams of star anise in capsules. Or swallow 300 milligrams of its essential oil. All are methods and doses recommended by Commission E.

Consumer Products Available

Fresh and powdered star anise is available in health food stores and ethnic food stores.

Potential Dangers

Commission E found no side effects, interaction with other drugs, or contraindications with star anise. *The PDR Family Guide to Natural Medicines & Healing Therapies* cautions consumers to "Be sure to avoid confusing star anise with the similar, but smaller, Japanese star anise, which is poisonous."

THYME

Thymus vulgaris

That sprig of thyme—a member of the mint family that's likely to adorn a garden or flavor soups and stews—is also good for healing. *Thymus vulgaris*, approved by Commission E, is domestic garden thyme. (Wild thyme, *Thymus sertpyllum*, is closely related and has a similar composition.) Both species of thyme grow wild in North America, Asia, and Europe.

Potential Health Benefits

Commission E endorses thyme to treat the symptoms of whooping cough and bronchitis (it's not considered a cure). Mainstream medicine evidently agrees; thyme is an ingredient in both Listerine and Vicks VapoRub.

Scientific Evidence

Chemists have identified the active ingredients in thyme oil as thymol and caracol. Both chemicals fight fungi and bacteria and are expectorants. Commission E doesn't cite clinical studies in its monograph, but thyme has a long history of safe use in Germany, and thyme-based medications are widely used there. Specifically, Commission E reviewed the properties of dried thyme leaves and flowers.

How to Use the Herb

Commission E recommends 1–2 grams of the herb for a cup of tea "several times a day as needed," or 1–2 grams of fluid extract 1 to 3 times per day. For wild thyme, which is slightly weaker than the garden variety, the commission recommends taking 6 grams per day. If you're unsure what type of thyme you have, try taking the smaller dose.

Consumer Products Available

Fresh thyme is sold in health food stores, herb shops, and supermarkets. Teas are available in the same outlets.

Potential Dangers

Commission E found no side effects, contraindications, or interactions with other drugs. Still, *The PDR Family Guide to Natural Medicines & Healing Therapies* advises: "Take no more than 10 grams of thyme daily." Note that the medicinal amounts recommended by Commission E are well below that ceiling, though they apply to dried leaves and flowers, not to other products such as thyme oil, which the commission did not evaluate.

TURMERIC ROOT

Curcuma longa

If you like spicy-hot Indian curries or bright-yellow American mustard, you probably like turmeric, the herb that gives these condiments their color. Like most culinary herbs, turmeric—which is grown in south Asia from India to Indonesia—also has medicinal qualities. It's a staple of traditional Indian Ayurvedic medicine, which uses preparations from the root of turmeric, a perennial herb. The powdered root is a prime ingredient in curry powder and is also called Indian saffron, although it doesn't come from the saffron plant.

Potential Health Benefits

Commission E endorses turmeric root as a treatment for dyspeptic conditions: upset stomach. Traditional and modern Asian healers have used turmeric much more widely, treating a range of conditions that the commission doesn't address: colds, worms, leprosy, headaches, leech bites.

Scientific Evidence

The active ingredient in turmeric powder is a chemical called curcumin, a natural antibiotic that helps retard food spoilage. Most scientific research on turmeric has been done in India, where animal studies suggest that turmeric attacks internal parasites and may help protect the liver against damage from alcohol. Other animal studies hint that turmeric, like its cousin ginger, may reduce cholesterol and slow untoward bloodclotting. A 1985 study published in the Western medical periodical *Cancer Letter* suggests that curcumin slows down the growth of lymphoma cancer cells.

One thing researchers in both the East and the West agree on is that turmeric stimulates the production of bile needed for digestion, adding to its utility in treating upset stomach.

How to Use the Herb

Commission E recommends an average daily dose of 1.5–3.0 grams of the powdered herb. Turmeric tea can be made by using 0.5–1.0 gram of powdered turmeric, steeping for 5 minutes, and straining; take the tea 2 to 3 times per day between meals. Herbal writer James A. Duke, Ph.D., recommends taking 1,200 milligrams of curcumin supplements daily in 3 doses of 400 milligrams each.

Consumer Products Available

Health food stores, pharmacies, and Asian food stores sell curcumin supplements as well as powdered turmeric. Duke advises curcumin-hungry consumers who also love curry to "go to an Indian grocery store and choose the yellowest variety of turmeric you can find." The yellower it is, he reasons, the more curcumin it contains.

Potential Dangers

Commission E found no side effects or interactions with other drugs, but does warn that turmeric shouldn't be used by anyone who has obstructed bile passages, and advises patients with gallstones to consult their doctors before using medicinal amounts of turmeric. Very large amounts of turmeric could irritate the stomach.

UVA URSI LEAF

Arctostaphylos uva-ursi

Native to Spain and known in England as bearberry, uva ursi is low-lying ground cover that grows in sandy soil in Europe and North America. North American Indians have long used it mixed with tobacco in a smoking mixture called kinnickinnik. The medicinal part of the plant are the leaves, which grow about an inch long and are dried before use.

Potential Health Benefits

Traditionally, and currently, uva ursi leaf is employed to treat urinary tract infections, and is approved for that purpose by Commission E. Uva ursi is also a key ingredient in herbal weight-loss formulas because it has a diuretic effect. Bear in mind that water-loss doesn't translate into long-term weight loss; more exercise and fewer calories are the most effective parts of any weight-loss plan.

Scientific Evidence

Uva ursi has an antibiotic effect, thanks to its active ingredient, arbutin, which is transformed in the urinary tract into hydroquinone. Uva ursi gets its diuretic properties from ursolic acid. Uva ursi is also high in astringent tannins. Another constituent, allantoin, is the active ingredient in skin creams such as Herpicin-L Cold Sore Lip Balm, but Commission E doesn't address this use of the herb and its derivatives.

How to Use the Herb

Commission E recommends average daily doses of 3 grams of the herb in 2/3 cup of water taken up to 4 times per day, or 400–840 milligrams of water-free arbutin. Uva ursi leaves must be soaked overnight to neutralize their harsh tannins. Several herbals point out that uva ursi works best when one's urine is alkaline; so, eat noncitrus fruits and vegetables if you're taking this drug, or use a little sodium bicarbonate to ensure alkalinity. Avoid acid-rich foods such as cranberry juice, citrus fruits, and sauerkraut. If you're using the herb to lose weight, be sure to replace the potassium that diuretics drive out of the body; eating bananas is an easy, tasty way of doing that.

Consumer Products Available

Health food stores and pharmacies stock teas in which uva ursi is included as an ingredient and, less frequently, sell uva ursi tea. Some health food stores sell powdered uva ursi supplements. *The PDR Family Guide to Natural Medicines & Healing Therapies* recommends taking capsules of 125–250 milligrams standardized to 20 percent arbutin 3 times a day.

Potential Dangers

Uva ursi shouldn't be used by lactating women or by pregnant women, as it can cause uterine contractions, or by children under 12. Commission E warns that the herb can cause nausea and vomiting in persons with sensitive stomachs. There are no known interactions with other drugs. The commission cautions that "Medications containing arbutin should not be taken for longer than a week or more than 5 times a year without consulting a physician."

VALERIAN ROOT
Valeriana officinalis

So highly regarded in medieval Europe that it was dubbed "all-heal," valerian is today used chiefly as a mild tranquilizer and as a natural sedative. Native to temperate Europe and Asia, it's also known as garden heliotrope. A perennial that can reach heights of five feet, valerian sprouts small, closely bunched flowers. It's the dried root that's used medicinally. When being dried, the root takes on a disagreeable odor likened to dirty gym socks (the whole, living garden plant smells fine). Valerian's scientific name is derived from the Latin word *valere*, translated as both "to be strong" and "to be healthy."

Potential Health Benefits

Commission E approves the dried roots of valerian as a treatment for restlessness and sleep disorders. Traditionally, valerian has been used to treat epilepsy. Some modern herbalists value its stress-busting properties for use against premenstrual syndrome and high blood pressure. Commission E didn't address these additional uses.

Scientific Evidence

Most scientific researchers attribute valerian's tranquilizing and sedative effects to chemicals found in its essential oil, called valepotriates, but that opinion isn't unanimous. In *Nature's Medicines*, author Joel L. Swerdlow, Ph.D., suggests that valerian's power may come from its gamma-aminobutyric acid (GABA), "a neurotransmitter that's thought to inhibit the brain's arousal system." In *Tyler's Honest Herbal*, Varro E. Tyler, Ph.D., submits that the exact triggering mechanism in valerian is unknown. While they may not agree on how valerian works, researchers agree that it does work. In a study of 128 insomniacs, patients who took 400 milligrams of valerian reported more dramatically improved sleep than patients taking a placebo; the herb worked better in women and test subjects under 40. Moreover, reports Andrew Weil, M.D., in a "placebo-controlled 1989 trial, 89 percent of those who ingested the herb reported improved sleep and 44 percent reported perfect sleep." Although the word valerian sounds similar to the prescription drug Valium, it isn't the same substance, as some people believe. Valium (diazepam) is synthesized in the laboratory; valerian is a plant.

How to Use the Herb

Commission E recommends 2–3 grams of the herb "one to several times a day" in rather foul-smelling tea. Additionally, the commission recommends ½–1 teaspoonful of tincture 1 to several times per day; and it recommends a liquid extract of 2–3 grams of valerian, also 1 to several times per day. In whatever form, valerian is best taken before bedtime. Be careful if you're driving or operating heavy machinery, as valerian depresses the central nervous system.

Consumer Products Available

Valerian tinctures, capsules, and teas are sold in health food stores and drugstores. Some supplements are standardized to specific amounts of valepotriates. Given the imperfect state of our knowledge, these formulations are educated guesses, not certainties. Make sure the product label says *Valeriana officinalis*. A related species, *Valerian edulis*, is sometimes sold, too, but it doesn't have as many of what are thought to be valerian's active constituents.

When looking for valerian supplements, check the label to make sure the Latin name is there and that it specifies *Valeriana officinalis*, the form of the plant approved by Commission E and believed by scientists to be the most effective variety. Also, the label should specify that the root was used; that's the most medicinally active part of the plant. All five valerian products I reviewed cited the root, but check for yourself when you're shopping. Commission E prefers valerian in tinctures and teas, and American health writer Andrew Weil, M.D., recommends a tincture: an alcohol-based solution. The only tincture I reviewed, Nature's Way Valerian Root, didn't carry the plant's Latin name on the product label. Other companies sold mostly soft capsules. One-a-Day Bedtime & Rest, a tablet, combines valerian with five other active ingredients, including kava, which Commission E approves separately as a sedative, plus the minerals calcium and magnesium. As with other combination products, this product may work fine, but there's less research behind it. The sale of such products seems to be predicated on the idea that if one herb is good for you, several herbs must be several times better, which is debatable.

Potential Dangers

Commission E found no contraindications, side effects, or known interactions with other drugs. Although valerian appears safe for most people, it can cause restlessness and heart palpitations in sensitive people. Don't combine valerian with Valium or other prescription drugs such as Elavil or Xanax. Taken by itself, valerian lacks the side effects often seen with prescription drugs and, unlike Valium, doesn't interfere with deep, REM dream sleep. Even so, many herbalists advise against long-term use (more than two weeks).

WATERCRESS

Nasturtium officinale

This peppery green plant, grown all over the world, gets its tingly quality from a key constituent: mustard oil. Long a favorite in salads and sandwiches, watercress also has medicinal qualities.

Potential Health Benefits

Commission E endorses watercress—specifically, the fresh or dried leaves and stems—to loosen phlegm and treat inflammation of the respiratory tract. Watercress compresses are used in Italy to treat arthritis, and homeopaths prescribe their customary minute doses to deal with a range of maladies that haven't been verified by the commission.

Scientific Evidence

Commission E puts the stamp of approval on watercress without citing scientific studies. *The PDR Family Guide to Natural Medicines & Healing Therapies* seconds Commission E, recommending watercress as a means of fighting cough and bronchitis. The PDR book credits watercress's medicinal powers to "mustard oil, a compound that flushes excess water from the body" and refers to unnamed researchers who "have also shown that the herb kills bacteria." It doesn't say which bacteria.

How to Use the Herb

Commission E recommends a daily dose of 4–6 grams of dried herb; 20–30 grams of fresh herb; or 60–150 grams of freshly pressed juice. Watercress tea can be made by pouring boiling water over ½ teaspoonful of crushed herb and steeping for 10 minutes.

Consumer Products Available

Fresh watercress is sold in supermarkets and other food stores. Dried watercress and teas are available in health food stores and groceries.

Potential Dangers

Commission E advises consumers to keep watercress away from children under four and rules out its use for anyone with ulcers or inflammatory kidney disease. Owing to the herb's high concentration of mustard oil, it can irritate the stomach.

WHITE WILLOW BARK

Salix alba

This native of central and southern Europe, now grown in temperate wetlands around the world, is widely recognized for its grace and beauty. It's not the long, slender leaves and hanging branches that are used medicinally, however, but the bark of the tree. Willow bark was used as a painkiller and anti-inflammatory drug in ancient Mesopotamia, in ancient China, and among Native Americans. The white willow is a source of salicin, which eventually led to the laboratory synthesis of aspirin.

Potential Health Benefits

Commission E recommends white willow bark as a medicine for diseases accompanied by fever, rheumatic ailments, inflammation, and headaches. In Asia, the bark is also employed to combat jaundice, a use not endorsed by Commission E.

Scientific Evidence

Salicin, which French and German chemists isolated in the 1820s, is the active pain- and inflammation-fighting chemical in white willow bark. The bark isn't as concentrated as laboratory aspirin, and thus not as strong, but it works in a similar way and doesn't upset the stomach as much as more-potent aspirin. Herbalists consider it to be a natural, gentle version of aspirin. Despite its similarity to aspirin, white willow bark hasn't been tested in scientific studies for efficacy in preventing heart attacks and strokes, as has aspirin (acetylsalicylis acid) in recent years.

How to Use the Herb

Commission E recommends an average daily dose of 60–120 milligrams of salicin, the active ingredient in either liquid or solid preparations. White willow bark can be taken in a tea, made by putting 1–2 teaspoonfuls of powdered bark in cold water, and then boiling the water and letting it steep for 5 minutes. Take the tea 3 to 5 times per day. The tea is bitter; adding honey can help it go down.

Consumer Products Available

White willow bark tea is sold in health food stores.

Potential Dangers

Although white willow bark hasn't been reported to cause aspirin-like side effects, herbalists recommend that pregnant women give it a pass and thus avoid the risk of birth defects. Similarly, the herb shouldn't be given to children under 16 who may be at risk for Reye's syndrome, a potentially fatal condition. It also shouldn't be taken with aspirin or by people with ulcers or other gastrointestinal conditions.

Witch Hazel Leaf and Bark

Hamamelis virginiana

This familiar member of the family medicine cabinet goes back to pre-Columbian times when Native Americans used witch hazel for a wide variety of ailments. A small tree or shrub native to the eastern United States and Canada, witch hazel is now widely grown, and is very popular in Europe. It's also known as winterbloom, for its yellow flowers, which blossom after the leaves drop off in the fall.

Potential Health Benefits

Commission E recommends both witch hazel leaf and bark for use against minor skin irritation and inflamed mucous membranes as well as means to shrink hemorrhoids and treat varicose veins. Some 1 million gallons of witch hazel water are sold every year in the United States, where it's made as a steam distillate. Witch hazel is also an ingredient in several popular American and German hemorrhoid preparations.

Scientific Evidence

Chemists have identified high tannin content—at least 4 percent, according to Commission E—in witch hazel. Commission E also credits witch hazel with anti-inflammatory powers and says it's locally hemostatic: that is, it slows down the flow of blood, which makes it useful for treating wounds. The commercial distilled witch hazel water sold in the United States—unlike the German brands reviewed by Commission E—contains virtually no tannins, prompting author Varro E. Tyler, Ph.D., to ascribe its astringent qualities to the 14 percent alcohol in the products. Health writer Michael Castleman counters that witch hazel water "does contain other chemicals with reported antiseptic anesthetic, astringent and anti-inflammatory action," although he doesn't name them. Tyler cites a 1997 study published in *Planta Medica* that found that some chemicals in witch hazel bark and leaves inhibit platelet-activities involved in inflammation. He also cites a 1996 study that suggests "strong antioxidant activity . . . may also play a role in witch hazel's anti-inflammatory effects."

How to Use the Herb

Commission E specifies these doses for external use: witch hazel water in virtually any amount as a rubbing liniment; for compresses and rinses, steep 5–10 grams of crushed witch hazel in 1 cup of water; for poultices, 20–30 percent in semisolid preparations. For internal use, the commission recommends suppositories 1 to 3 times per day.

Consumer Products Available

Witch hazel distillates are available in supermarkets and pharmacies. The powdered herb is sold in health food stores. Witch hazel is also frequently an ingredient in commercial gels, ointments, and suppositories.

Potential Dangers

Witch hazel—so long as it isn't swallowed, and it's not supposed to be—is very safe. There are no known contraindications, side effects, or drug interactions.

YARROW
Achillea millefolium

The *Achillea* in yarrow's Latin name refers to Achilles, Homer's legendary Greek hero, who supposedly staunched the bleeding of his soldiers' wounds in the Trojan War by brushing them with yarrow. In line with this, yarrow is also known as woundwort. Growing in southern and eastern Europe and parts of Asia, yarrow has fern-like leaves and stalks topped with clusters of tiny pink or white flowers. It's botanically related to daisies, marigolds, and dandelions. Commission E evaluated the fresh and dried above-ground parts of the plant, harvested in flowering season.

Potential Health Benefits

Commission E found yarrow useful for treating loss of appetite, mild discomfort of the gastrointestinal tract, and upset stomach when used internally. The commission recommends yarrow to be used externally, in a sitz bath, for "painful, cramp-like conditions of psychosomatic origin in the lower part of the female pelvis." The commission didn't address traditional, and decidedly nonpsychosomatic, uses of yarrow in healing wounds, or new ones suggested in studies for treating hepatitis.

Scientific Evidence

Commission E's monograph on yarrow ascribes many virtues to the plant: antibacterial, antispasmotic, and astringent. Without citing other sources, the commission also describes yarrow as choleretic—that is, it stimulates the liver to increase the production of bile, which aids in digestion. A study conducted in India and published in 1976 in the *Indian Journal of Medical Research* finds yarrow to have value in treating liver diseases—chiefly, hepatitis. This is an interesting lead for additional research that may well be needed in the West and elsewhere.

How to Use the Herb

For internal use, Commission E recommends 4.5 grams of yarrow herb, or 3 grams of yarrow flower. To make tea, put 2 grams of dried yarrow in boiling water and steep 10–15 minutes. For external use, 100 grams (20 teaspoonfuls) of dried yarrow in 5 gallons of warm water is just right for a sitz bath.

Consumer Products Available

Dried yarrow herb and flower and yarrow teas are sold in health food stores. Dried yarrow in capsule form is available in health food stores and drugstores.

Potential Dangers

Yarrow causes allergies in some people, producing a nasty rash. Commission E reports no known drug interactions or contraindications. However, the *Prevention* magazine book *Nature's Medicines* advises pregnant women to steer clear of medicinal quantities of yarrow.

PART 2

THE DUBIOUS DOZEN

Commission E placed 126 herbs and six fixed-combination herbal preparations on its unapproved list.

Making the unapproved list doesn't necessarily mean that these herbal medicines have no value for anyone, ever. Rather, it means that the experts on the commission didn't see hard evidence that the herbs worked in the ways they're supposed to, or that the advantages of using them clearly outweigh the risks. Some herbs are harmless in themselves but won't cure you; others may actually sabotage your health.

Commission E sometimes approves one part of a plant and not another. For example, it okayed a standardized extract of milk thistle fruit but nixed medicinal use of the whole herb on the grounds that traditional claims for its value in treating jaundice and pleurisy, among other maladies, are unproven.

Here's a selection of herbs that Commission E, for one reason or another, put on its unapproved list. Some may surprise you.

BORAGE

Borage officinalis

Borage, an annual herb valued as a mood-enhancer as far back as 2,000 years ago, was judged high-risk by Commission E, which evaluated the flower and the whole herb. The commission noted that borage contains toxic pyrrolizidine alkaloids (PA), which can harm the liver and have caused cancer in laboratory animals. The commission's evaluation can be extended to borage oil, which is sold in North American health food stores to treat coughs and lighten bad moods.

Some American health writers disagree with the commission. James A. Duke, Ph.D., praises borage for its high content of gamma-linolenic acid (GLA), "a substance useful in treating a number of disorders, including . . . autoimmune disorders . . . diabetes, and migraines." The *Prevention* magazine book *Nature's Medicines* also writes approvingly of the GLA in borage, citing a scientific study in which a group of chronic dermatitis patients who took 272 milligrams of borage oil twice per day for 12 weeks got much greater relief from itching and blistering than did a placebo group.

Nevertheless, many herb authorities think that borage isn't worth the risk. *New York Times* health writer Jane E. Brody put borage on an "herbs to avoid" list in 1999. Varro E. Tyler, Ph.D., red-flags borage for its unsaturated PA content, cautioning that "chronic consumption of either the borage plant or its seed oil should be carried out only under medical supervision, unless the products are certified free of UPAs."

DAMIANA LEAF AND HERB

Turnera diffusa

Although damiana—commonly sold in North American health food stores as Mexican damiana—has a huge reputation as an aphrodisiac, especially for women, Commission E could find no justification for that reputation. The commission doesn't think that using damiana will hurt you, just that it will disappoint you.

Some herbal writers beg to disagree. In their book *Sex Herbs*, authors Beth Ann Petro Roybal and Gayle Skowronski say that this small Mexican shrub "provides needed oxygen to the genital area." Citing the experience of happy herbal fans, they conclude "You would be hard-pressed to find a more useful herb today."

However, according to some other herbal authorities, all those damiana pills, extracts, and teas sold in health food stores and drugstores are a waste of money. Varro E. Tyler, Ph.D., for one, declares flat out: "No constituent responsible for claims of damiana as an aphrodisiac has ever been identified."

EPHEDRA (MA HUANG)

Ephedra sinica

This book singles out one herb—sarsaparilla—that Commission E judged unapproved, but we put it on our list of "Herbs That Work." Here we're doing the opposite: that is, we're taking one herb that the commission approved (for treating asthma, colds, and flu) and putting it on our "Dubious Dozen" list. That herb is ephedra. The weight of evidence from many sources suggests that self-medicating with ephedra—known in Chinese medicine as ma huang—isn't worth the risk.

A spiky evergreen shrub native to China and Mongolia, ma huang has been used in traditional Chinese medicine for 5,000 years. In modern times, Japanese kamikaze fighter pilots took megadoses of ephedra to get their metabolism racing. Today, over-the-counter ephedra drugs are very popular, both for boosting athletic performance and for promoting weight loss. Both actions are attributed to the herb's active ingredient, ephedrine, which stimulates the central nervous system. (*Note:* The American plant known as Mormon tea, *E. nevadensis*, is a different species of ephedra, and most herbalists don't attribute dramatic physiological effects to it.)

There are many problems with the popular Asian form of ephedra. It can trigger dangerously high blood pressure and cause heart palpitations, dizziness, and insomnia. It's especially risky for persons with hypertension, glaucoma, thyroid disorders, diabetes, and heart disease. Jane E. Brody, a *New York Times* health writer, points out that ephedra "contains cardiac toxins resulting in dozens of deaths." Varro E. Tyler, Ph.D., considers ephedra an effective decongestant when used in small doses but warns, "the side effects indicated render its indiscriminate use highly inadvisable. . . ."

In our enthusiastically self-medicating society—which is, additionally, a society obsessed with weight—that's a real concern. Quick fixes rarely fix anything.

HIBISCUS

Hibiscus sabdariffa

Hibiscus—a relative of marshmallow herb—produces very pretty flowers that don't do a darn thing medicinally, in Commission E's opinion. Hibiscus flower preparations are used internally to restore lost appetite, to dissolve phlegm, as a laxative, and for circulatory problems. Hibiscus does have a mild laxative effect, and it won't hurt you—but that's about it, according to the commission. Better to grow hibiscus in the garden and admire its lovely red and yellow flowers than waste your time and money by consuming them.

HYSSOP

Hyssopus officinalis

Commission E also cast a cold eye on hyssop, the source of an herbal oil and tea sold in health food stores as a treatment for colds, chest and lung ailments, a stimulant to circulation, aid for digestion, treatment for menstrual discomfort, heart problems, even pain in the eye. If hyssop could help all these conditions, it would be a panacea, but the commission says it can't. "There is no objection to the use of hyssop herb below 5 percent," as a flavoring agent in tea, the commission decided, but beyond that, no.

KELP

Laminaria stipites

Kelp, long strands of brown seaweed, algae commonly found along ocean shorelines, is a key ingredient in Japanese cuisine. Its high iodine content is alleged to be useful for treating a wide range of conditions and maladies. Among the uses that kelp—dried, powdered, and pressed into tablets—is supposed to help alleviate are constipation, gallstones, obesity, arthritis, skin diseases, and thyroid disorders. Commission E, focusing on thyroid therapy, ruled that iodine doses above 150 micrograms per day could cause allergic reactions or make hypothyroidism even worse. Below 150 micrograms per day, kelp containing iodine isn't proven effective for the many things it's supposed to help. Either way, the commission found kelp of dubious medicinal value. Moreover, kelp can be contaminated by polluted seas. A 1995 report in *Environmental Health Perspectives* found that kelp and other seafoods consumed by Canadian Inuit (Eskimos) was high in both toxic cadmium and lead.

LEMONGRASS (CITRONELLA)

Cymbopogon species

Relax, you can still keep enjoying lemongrass in Thai and Vietnamese cuisine. It's the medicinal uses of the plant and its oil that Commission E found lacking. The commission evaluated lemongrass and its oil from a variety of sources: Sri Lanka, the West Indies, and the Indonesian island of Java. The above-ground plant and its oil are claimed to be effective for treating digestive disorders, muscle pain, neuralgia, colds, and "various nervous disorders." The commission wasn't impressed, deciding that convincing documentation is lacking. Using lemongrass herb and oil for taste and aroma is fine, but don't expect medical cures. Citronella, another name for Asian lemongrass, is considered effective as a source of insect repellent, an important application in the buggy tropics.

OLIVE OIL

Olive oleum

Relax, you can keep enjoying olive oil in Italian and other cuisines. Just don't think of it as powerful medicine. While olive oil has many champions who favor it as one of the heart-healthy seed oils, Commission E evaluated it as a wide-ranging remedy. Olive oil has been used in Europe in ointments to treat tinnitus (ringing in the ear), to prevent or erase stretch marks during pregnancy, and in gelatin capsules for firming up the breasts. The commission found no solid documentation for these uses. Additionally, it warned against attempting to treat gallstones by ingesting olive oil, another traditional therapy. Actually, olive oil induces cramps in people with gallstones.

OREGANO

Origanum vulgare

Keep relaxing—oregano is still fine for sprinkling on pizza. The oil in oregano leaves does help loosen phlegm in the lungs and ease spasmodic coughing. However, Commission E could find no proof of oregano's claimed value in treating urinary tract disorders, painful menstruation, arthritis, or abdominal diseases—all traditional uses. Oregano is in no way harmful, but the commission report states "The claimed efficacy for this herb has not been documented."

ROSE HIPS

Rosa canina

Rose hips won't hurt you, but they will lighten your pocketbook if you expect them to treat gallstones, strengthen the kidneys, combat arthritis, or improve bowel disorders. Rose hips aren't even very good sources of vitamin C, the commission declared, and what vitamin C content they do have deteriorates rapidly in storage. (For more on uses of rose hips, see the "Herbs That Work" entry on rose flower.)

SAFFRON

Crocus sativus

As a culinary herb, the smooth, savory qualities in saffron make it hard to beat. However, its alleged medicinal qualities are dubious, indeed. Commission E found no evidence for saffron's traditional use as a sedative and treatment for spasms and asthma. Additionally, the commission worries that saffron poses health risks. While a daily therapeutic dose of 1.5 grams is safe, as little as 5 grams per day of saffron, the commission notes, can trigger "pitch-black necrosis of the nose . . . and severe collapse with uremia." Some American herbal writers contend that saffron has a protective effect on the heart, but Commission E doesn't address that point.

YOHIMBE

Pausinystalia yohimbe

Another herb . . . another aphrodisiac debunked. The bark of yohimbe, a West African tree, is said to boost male and female sex drive by increasing blood flow to the genitals. Yohimbe can be purchased in capsules, tablets, extracts, and drops sold in health food stores and drugstores. Commission E was decidedly unmoved by this herbal Viagra, finding insufficient documentation for its value and more than sufficient documentation for its risks. The commission notes that the dried bark can cause nervous exhaustion, tremors, sleeplessness, and other signs of being wired, without the hoped-for benefits. Beth Ann Petro Roybal and Gayle Skowronski are similarly cautious about yohimbe in their book *Sex Herbs*, noting its many side effects while not dismissing it outright. Varro E. Tyler, Ph.D., writing in *Tyler's Honest Herbal*, concludes that the herb warrants further study but allows that with the emergence of Viagra, it probably won't happen.

Appendix

If you contemplate using an herbal remedy, consult with a physician and talk to a health care provider familiar with herbal remedies and/or a trained herbalist to find out how it might impact your health. The following lists are guidelines for you to consider:

Drugs to Avoid

In Children Under 12

Aloe (internally)
Camphor
Eucalyptus leaf and oil
Fennel oil
Horseradish (children under 4)
Mint oil (external)
Mistletoe berries
Peppermint oil (external)
Rhubarb root
Watercress (children under 4)
White willow bark (children under 16 who may be at risk for Reye's syndrome)

When You Have AIDS

Echinacea pallida root
Mistletoe

When You Are a Diabetic

Echinacea purpurea (injectable)
Marshmallow
Psyllium seed, black
Psyllium seed, blonde

When You Have Gallbladder Disease

Chicory
Dandelion
Devil's claw root
Ginger
Haronga bark and leaf
Mint oil
Peppermint leaves and oil
Turmeric (medicinal amounts)

When You Have Heart Disease

Belladonna
Ginseng
Goldenrod
Hawthorn leaf with flower (certain cardiac
        conditions, please check with a physician)
Horehound herb
Horsetail
Licorice
Parsley (medicinal amounts)

When You Have Kidney Disease

Goldenrod
Horsetail
Juniper berry

Licorice
Parsley (medicinal amounts)
Sarsaparilla
Watercress

When You Have Liver Problems

Eucalyptus leaf and oil
Haronga bark and leaf
Licorice
Mint oil
Peppermint oil

When You Have Multiple Sclerosis

Echinacea pallida root
Echinacea purpurea

When You Have Prostate Problems

Belladonna

When Pregnant or Nursing

Aloe (internally)
Black cohosh root
Cinnamon oil and bark
Comfrey herb and leaf
Echinacea purpurea (injectable)
Fennel oil
Fenugreek (use with caution)
Ginger (challenged by some experts)
Juniper berry
Kava kava
Licorice

Mistletoe

Parsley (medicinal amounts)

Rhubarb

Rosemary (medicinal amounts)

Sage (essential oil and alcoholic
    extracts)

Uva ursi

White willow bark

Yarrow

When You Have Ulcers

Cinnamon oil

Cola nut

Devil's claw root

Horseradish

Watercress

White willow bark

Drug Interactions

Belladonna and antidepressants

Cola nut and antidepressants

Garlic and anticoagulants

Gingko and blood-thinners, including aspirin

Horse chestnut seed and blood-thinners

Kava kava and alcohol, barbiturates

Sarsaparilla and hypnotics

St. John's wort and alcohol

St. John's wort and antidepressants and tranquilizers

St. John's wort and HIV medication

Valerian and tranquilizers and antidepressants

Interactions by Drug or Other Substance

Alcohol and kava kava
Amantadine and belladonna leaf and root
Antiarrythmic agents and aloe
Barbiturates and kava kava
Caffeine-containing beverages and cola nut
Cardiac glycosides and aloe
Corticosteroids and aloe
Digitalis glycosides and licorice root
Licorice root and aloe
MAO inhibitors and brewer's yeast
Psychoanaleptic drugs and cola nut
Psychopharmacological agents and kava kava
Quinidine and belladonna leaf and root
Thiazide diuretics and aloe and licorice root
Tricyclic antidepressants and belladonna leaf and root
Urine-acidifying agents and uva ursi leaf

Herbs that Affect Drug Absorption or Increase Sensitivities to Other Drugs

Brewer's yeast
Eucalyptus oil
Flaxseed
Licorice root
Marshmallow leaf and root
Psyllium seed, blonde
Rhubarb root
Sarsaparilla
Uva ursi
White willow bark

Herbs Not to Be Taken Over a Lengthy Period of Time

Aloe
Bilberry fruit
Black cohosh root
Blackberry leaf
Comfrey herb and leaf
Echinacea
Fennel oil and seed
Ginkgo biloba leaf extract
Ginseng root
Hawthorn leaf with flower
Kava kava
Licorice root
Paprika (externally)
Psyllium seed, blonde
Rhubarb root
Uva ursi
Valerian

GLOSSARY

Analgesic: a pain-killer

Anaphylactic shock: an allergic response that triggers difficulty breathing and sharply lowers blood-pressure

Antibacterial: destroying bacteria or slowing their growth

Anticoagulant: preventing clotting of the blood

Antiseptic: inhibiting the growth of infectious organisms

Antispasmodic: preventing spasms

Aromatic bitter: a bitter used as a flavoring agent in food or medication

Astringent: an agent causing contraction

Bitter: a bitter-tasting liquid that stimulates the appetite by increasing saliva and gastric juices

Bitter principles: constituents with a bitter taste, caused by the presence of alkaloids

Carcinogen: a substance that causes cancer

Catarrh: term for inflammation of the mucous membranes, especially in the respiratory system

Choleretic: an agent that stimulates the liver to increase the production of bile

Decoction: a liquid made by boiling herbs in water for a long time, as much as 20 minutes, that is consumed like tea

Demulcent: an agent that soothes irritation of the mucous membrane; usually an oily substance

Diuretic: an agent that stimulates urine output; many things do this, including coffee

Dosage: the amount of a medicine

Dose: the amount of a medicine and how often it's taken

Dry extract: extract of a plant material in which the solvent has evaporated, leaving a solid base

Dyspepsia: indigestion

Eczema: inflammation of the skin

Edema: an abnormal accumulation of liquid in tissue, such as in the legs or feet

Electrolyte: a substance in liquid solution that conducts an electrical current

Emetic: a substance that induces vomiting

Essential oil: volatile terpene derivatives that impart taste and aroma

Expectorant: promoting the liquidization of mucous that can then be expelled

Flavonoids: naturally occurring compounds in plants that act as antioxidants and anti- inflammatory agents

Flower: the reproductive structure of some seed-bearing plants

Fluid extract: a concentrated mix of water and alcohol in which 1 milliliter is equivalent to 1 gram of the original plant material

Folium: Latin for *leaf*

Fruit: the matured ovary of flowering plants

Fungistatic: inhibiting the growth of fungi

Genus: the first word in two-word Latin designations of plants, referring to a group of species exhibiting similar characteristics

High-density lipoprotein: so-called good cholesterol that doesn't accumulate in blood vessels

Homeopathy: a system of medicine founded by the German physician Samuel Hahnemann in which minute amounts of drugs are used that, in larger doses, would produce symptoms of the disease being treated

Hybrid: the offspring of genetically different parents or stock in animal and plants

Infusion: a liquid made by immersing herbs without boiling in order to extract soluble elements or active principles

Irrigation therapy: washing out a cavity or wound with a liquid, sometimes an herbal tea

Isoflavone: plant component that shares similarities with the female sex hormone estrogen

Leaf: a photosynthetic organ, usually green, on the stem of a plant

Liniment: on ointment

Linoleic acid: a polyunsaturated fat that lowers blood cholesterol

Lipid: fat-soluble substances derived from animal or vegetable cells, insoluble in water but soluble in organic solvents, oily to the touch, including fats, oils, waxes, and sterols

Low-density lipoprotein: so-called bad cholesterol, implicated in clogging of the arteries

Mucilage: a gelatinous plant substance mixed with water and used to soothe irritated mucous membranes

Ointment: a semisolid preparation used for topical application to the skin

Perennial: a plant living for two or more years

Poultice: a soft mass prepared by adding water to plant materials and applying to the skin

Pungent principles: essential oils that convey odor

Radix: Latin for *root*

Rhizome: the underground stem of a plant, with leaves growing from the top and roots from the bottom

Root: the absorbing and anchoring underground organ of a plant, usually growing downward

Seed: the mature ovule of seed plants

Sitz bath: an immersion bath, from the German *sitzen*, to sit

Soporific: sleep-inducing

Stem: a supporting and conducting plant organ, growing upward

Synergistic: the action of two or more agents exceeding the sum of their parts

Tea: an infusion made by pouring boiling water over plant material (usually leaves), steeping, and drinking

Tincture: a solution made by immersing herbs in alcohol and taken as medicine, usually in drops

Tonic: a mixture of herbs in alcohol, taken as a means of restoring health and vigor

Topical application: smoothing on the skin, as in an ointment or salve

Volatile oil: easily evaporated terpene derivatives that impart taste and aroma

WEIGHTS AND MEASURES CHART

METRIC WEIGHT

kg (kilo)	one kilogram	=1,000 grams
cg	one centigram	=0.01 grams
mg	one milligram	=0.001 grams
mcg	one microgram	=0.0001 grams

METRIC CONVERSION CHART

WHEN YOU KNOW	MULTIPLY BY	TO FIND
	Volume	
liters	1.06	quarts
liters	.026	gallons
teaspoons	4.93	milliliters
tablespoons	14.78	milliliters
fluid ounces	29.57	milliliters
cups	.24	liters
pints	.47	liters
quarts	3.79	liters

WHEN YOU KNOW	MULTIPLY BY	TO FIND
	Mass and Weight	
grams	.035	ounce
kilograms	2.21	pounds
ounces	28.35	grams
pounds	.45	kilograms

WHEN YOU KNOW	MULTIPLY BY	TO FIND
	Volume	
milliliters	.20	tps
milliliters	.06	tbs
milliliters	.03	fl ozs
liters	4.23	cups
liters	2.12	pints

BIBLIOGRAPHY

Armstrong, David. *The Insider's Guide to Health Foods.* New York: Bantam, 1984.

Armstrong, David and Armstrong, Elizabeth Metzger. *The Great American Medicine Show.* New York: Prentice Hall Press, 1991.

Blumenthal, Mark, senior editor. *The Complete German Commission E Monographs: Therapeutic Guide to Herbal Medicines.* Austin, TX: American Botanic Council, 1998.

Castleman, Michael. *The Healing Herbs.* Emmaus, PA: Rodale Press, 1991.

Duke, James A., Ph.D. *Dr. Duke's Essential Herbs.* Emmaus, PA: Rodale Books, 1999.

Evennett, Karen. *Garlic: The Natural Remedy.* Berkeley, CA: Ulysses Press, 1998.

Foster, Steven and Tyler, Varro E., Ph.D. *Tyler's Honest Herbal.*, fourth edition. Binghamton, NY: Haworth Herbal Press, 1999.

Karch, Steven B., M.D. *The Consumer's Guide to Herbal Medicine.* Hauppauge, NY: Advanced Research Press, 1999.

Malesky, Gale. *Nature's Medicines.* Emmaus, PA: Rodale Press, 1999.

Roybal, Beth Ann Petro and Skowronski, Gayle. *Sex Herbs.* Berkeley, CA: Ulysses Press, 1999.

Selby, Anne. *The Ancient and Healing Art of Chinese Herbalism.* Berkeley, CA: Ulysses Press, 1998.

_____. *The PDR Family Guide to Natural Medicines &* *Healing Therapies.* New York: Three Rivers Press, 1999.

INDEX

Aches and pains
  and comfrey, 32
  and eucalyptus, 45
  and horseradish, 77
  and mint oil, 96
  and paprika, 107
  and peppermint, 112
Acne problems, and brewer's
  yeast, 16, 17
AIDS/HIV
  and aloe, 4
  contraindications, 183
  and echinacea, 40–41
Aloe, 3–4
American Botanical Council,
  xii–xiii
  on brewer's yeast, 17
  on ginger, 57
  on rosemary leaf, 133
Angina, and hawthorn, 69
Anise seed, 5–6
Anxiety, stress, and restlessness
  and chamomile flower, 22, 23
  and ginseng, 62
  and hops, 71
  and kava kava, 83
  and lavender, 85
  and St. John's wort, 141

Appetite problems
  and brewer's yeast, 16
  and chicory, 24
  and cinnamon bark, 26
  and dandelion, 34
  and devil's claw root, 36
  and fenugreek seed, 49
  and horehound herb, 73
  and juniper berry, 81
  and onion, 104
  and orange peel, 106
  and paprika, 107
  and pollen, 116
  and yarrow, 163
Asia, and herbal medicines, xiv
Aspirin
  and gingko biloba, 60
  compared to white willow
    bark, 159
Asthma, and onion, 104

Bearberry (uva ursi leaf),
  151–52
Belladonna, 7–8
Bilberry fruit, 9–10
Bile and bile duct problems
  and belladonna, 7
  and chicory, 24

and cinnamon, 26
and dandelion, 34
and devil's claw root, 36
and haronga, 67
and horehound herb, 73
and peppermint, 112
and radish, 126
and turmeric root, 150
and yarrow, 163
Bitter orange peel, 11
Black cohosh root, 12–13
Blackberry leaf, 14–15
Bladder stones
    and goldenrod, 65
    and horsetail herb, 79
    and juniper berry, 81
Bloating. *See* Flatulence and gas
    problems
Blonz, Ed, on licorice root,
    90
Blood pressure. *See* High blood
    pressure problems
Borage, 170
Bottle brush (horsetail herb),
    79–80
Breastfeeding, contraindications,
    185–86
Breathing problems
    and camphor, 18
    and eucalyptus, 45
    and horseradish, 77
    See also Respiratory tract in-
        flammation
Brewer's yeast, 16–17
Brody, Jane
    on borage, 170
    on ephedra, 172

Bronchitis. *See* Colds, flu, and
    bronchitis
Bruisewort (comfrey), 32–33
Buckeye (horse chestnut seed),
    75–76
Burns
    and aloe, 3
    and St. John's wort, 141
Butter rose (primrose), 118–19

Camphor, 18–19
Cancer
    and anise seed, 5
    and flaxseed, 51
    and garlic, 54
    and mistletoe, 98
    and turmeric root, 149
Caraway seed, 20–21
Castleman, Michael
    on anise seed, 6
    on blackberry leaf, 14
    on marshmallow, 91
    on paprika, 108
    on parsley, 111
    on rhubarb root, 129
    on rose flower, 131
    on rosemary leaf, 133
    on witch hazel, 161–62
Cayenne, 107–109
Chamomile flower, 22–23
Chicory, 24–25
Children, contraindications, 183.
    See also specific herbs
Cholesterol problems
    and brewer's yeast, 16
    and fenugreek seed, 49–50
    and garlic, 53

and psyllium seed, 120–21
and turmeric root, 141
Chronic fatigue syndrome, and
ginseng, 62
Cinnamon bark, 26–27
Circulation, local
and camphor, 18
and eucalyptus, 45
and rosemary leaf, 132
Circulation problems
and ginkgo biloba, 58
and horse chestnut seed, 75
and onion, 104
Cirrhosis, and milk thistle fruit,
93
Citronella (lemongrass), 177
Cloves, 28–29
Cola nut, 30–31
Colds, flu, and bronchitis
and anise seed, 5
and camphor, 18
and echinacea, 40
and eucalyptus, 45
and fennel, 47
and horehound, 73
and licorice root, 89
and mint oil, 96
and paprika, 107
and plantain, 114–15
and rose flower, 130–31
and star anise seed, 145
See also Coughing problems;
Respiratory tract inflam-
mation
Comfrey, 32–33
Commission E, xi–xiii, xiv. See
also specific herbs

Concentration problems
and cola nut, 30
and ginseng, 62
Constipation problems
and flaxseed, 51
and psyllium seed, 120, 122
Contraindications, 183–86. See
also specific herbs
Conversion (metric) chart, 193
Coughing problems
and camphor, 18
and horehound herb, 73
and mullein flower, 102
and star anise seed, 145
and watercress, 157
Cowslip (primrose), 118–19
Cramps, menstrual, and yarrow,
163
Cramps, stomach, and star anise
seed, 145
Cramps, and yarrow, 163
Cure-all (lemon balm), 87–88

Damiana leaf and herb, 171
Dandelion, 34–35
Dangers, 183–88. See also specific
herbs
Deadly nightshade (belladonna),
7–8
Dementia, and gingko biloba, 58,
59
Dental problems
and cloves, 28
and echinacea, 40
Depression
and ginseng, 62
and St. John's wort, 141, 144

Devil's claw root, 36–37
Diabetes
    and aloe, 3–4
    and brewer's yeast, 16
    contraindications, 184
    and fenugreek seed, 49–50
    and marshmallow, 91
    and psyllium seed, 123
    and sage, 134–35
Diarrhea problems
    and blackberry leaf, 14
    and brewer's yeast, 16, 17
    and psyllium seed, 120,
        122
Digestion problems. *See* Stomach
    problems
Dill seed, 38–39
Diuretics and fluid retention
    and cola nut, 30
    and dandelion, 34
    and goldenrod, 65
    and horsetail herb, 79
    and juniper berry, 81
    and parsley, 110
    and sarsaparilla, 136
    and uva ursi leaf, 151
Dosages. *See specific herbs*
Drug absorption problems, 187.
    See also specific herbs
"Dubious dozen" (unapproved
    herbs), 169–82
Duke, James A.
    on borage, 170
    on bilberry fruit, 9, 10
    on echinacea, 40–41
    on onion, 104
    on pumpkin seed, 124

on saw palmetto berry,
    140
on turmeric root, 150

Echinacea, 40–44
Energy and fatigue problems
    and cola nut, 30–31
    and ginseng, 62–64
    and sarsaparilla, 136
Ephedra, 172–73
Epilepsy, and valerian root,
    153
Eucalyptus, 45–46
Eye problems
    and belladonna, 7
    and bilberry fruit, 9
    and fennel, 47
    and gingko biloba, 58
    and onion, 104

Fairy cap (primrose), 118–19
Fatigue. *See* Energy and fatigue
    problems
Felt wort (mullein flower),
    102–103
Fennel, 47–48
Fenugreek, 49–50
Fever
    and anise seed, 5
    and white willow bark, 159
Flatulence and gas problems
    and caraway seeds, 20
    and cinnamon bark, 26
    and horehound herb, 73
    and lavender, 85
    and lemon balm, 87
    and mint oil, 96

Flaxseed, 51–52
Flu. *See* Colds, flu, and bronchitis
Flying (airplane) problems, and
　echinacea, 40, 41

Gallbladder disease, contraindica-
　tions, 184
Garden heliotrope (valerian root),
　153–56
Garlic, 53–55
Gas. *See* Flatulence and gas
　problems
Gastrointestinal problems. *See*
　Diarrhea problems; Stomach
　problems
German chamomile flower, 22–23
Germany, and herbal medicine,
　xi–xiii, xiv. *See also specific herbs*
Ginger, 56–57
Ginkgo biloba, 58–61
Ginseng, 62–64
Goldenrod, 65–66

Haronga, 67–68
Hawthorn, 69–70
Headaches
　and paprika, 108
　and peppermint, 113
　and white willow bark, 159
Healing problems, and comfrey,
　32. *See also* Wounds and
　wound healing
Heart disease
　and chamomile flower, 22
　contraindications, 184
Heart palpitations, and mother-
　wort, 100

Heartwort (motherwort),
　100–101
Hemorrhoids, and witch hazel, 161
Hepatitis
　and milk thistle fruit, 93
　and yarrow, 163–64
Herb, defined, xii
Herbal medicines, ix–xiv
　approved, 3–164
　Power 8, xiii, 40–44, 53–55,
　　58–61, 62–64, 93–95,
　　138–40, 141–44, 153–56
　purchasing, xiv
　unapproved, 169–82
　See also specific herbs
Herpes simplex virus
　and licorice root, 89
　and mistletoe, 102
　and mullein flower, 102
Hibiscus, 174
High blood pressure problems
　and cinnamon, 26
　and garlic, 53
　and hawthorn, 69
　and mistletoe, 98
　and onion, 104
　and parsley, 110
　and sarsaparilla, 136
　and valerian root, 153
HIV. *See* AIDS/HIV
Hops, 71–72
Horehound herb, 73–74
Horse chestnut seed, 75–76
Horse willow (horsetail herb),
　79–80
Horseradish, 77–78
Horsetail herb, 79–80

Houndbane (horehound herb),
  73–74
Huckleberry (bilberry), 9–10
Hyssop, 174

Indian saffron (turmeric root),
  149–50
Indigestion. *See* Stomach problems
Infections and inflammation
  and anise seed, 5
  and chamomile flower, 22
  and devil's claw root, 36
  and echinacea, 41
  and fenugreek seed, 49
  and garlic, 53
  and white willow bark, 159
  and witch hazel, 161–62
Insomnia. *See* Sleeping problems
Interactions, 186–87. *See also spe-*
  cific herbs
Irritable bowel syndrome
  and mint oil, 96
  and psyllium seed, 120

Japanese star anise, 146
Juniper berry, 81–82

Karch, Steven B.
  on anise seed, 5
  on caraway seed, 20
  on chamomile flower, 22–23
  on Commission E, xii
  on devil's claw root, 36
  on fenugreek seed, 41
  on lavender, 85
  on primrose, 118
Kava kava, 83–84

Kelp, 176
Kidney problems
  contraindications, 184–85
  and goldenrod, 65
  and horsetail herb, 79
  and juniper berry, 81
  and parsley, 110
Knitbone (comfrey), 32–33
Koch, Heinrich, on garlic, 54
Kola. *See* Cola nut

Lavender, 85–86
Lawson, Larry, on garlic, 54
Laxatives
  and aloe, 3, 4
  and rhubarb root, 128
  and sarsaparilla, 136
Lemon balm, 87–88
Lemongrass, 177
Licorice root, 89–90
Liver problems
  contraindications, 185
  and milk thistle fruit, 93
Lydia Pinkham's Vegetable
  Compound, 12

Ma huang (ephedra), 172–73
Marshmallow, 91–92
Mayflower (hawthorn), 69–70
Melissa (lemon balm), 87–88
Memory problems, and gingko
  biloba, 58
Menstrual problems
  and black cohosh root, 12–13
  and parsley, 110
  and valerian root, 153
  and yarrow, 163

Metric conversion chart, 193
Mexican damiana, 171
Milk thistle fruit, 93–95
Mint oil, 96–97
Mistletoe, 98–99
Motherwort, 100–101
Motion sickness, and ginger, 56–57
Mullein flower, 102–103
Multiple sclerosis, contraindications, 185
Muscle pain. *See* Aches and pains

Nausea, and ginger, 56–57
Neuralgia (nerve inflammation), and peppermint, 112

Olive oil, 178
Onion, 104–105
Orange peel, 106
Orange peel, bitter, 11
Oregano, 179
Overdose information. *See specific herbs*

Pain problems, and devil's claw root, 36. *See also* Aches and pains
Paprika, 107–109
Parsley, 110–11
Pepper, red, 107–109
Peppermint, 112–13
Peppermint oil, 96–97
Perspiration problems, and sage, 134
Plantain, 114–15
Plantain (psyllium seed), 120–21
Pollen, 116–17

Power 8 herbs, xiii
echinacea, 40–44
garlic, 53–55
ginkgo biloba, 58–61
ginseng, 62–64
milk thistle, 93–95
saw palmetto berry, 138–40
St. John's wort, 141–44
valerian root, 153–56
Pregnancy, contraindications, 185–86
Primrose, 118–19
Prostate problems
contraindications, 185
and pumpkin seed, 124
and saw palmetto berry, 138, 140
Psoriasis, and sarsaparilla, 136
Psyllium seed, 120–23
black, 120–21
blond, 122–23
Pumpkin seed, 124–25

Radish, 126–27
Red pepper, 107–109
Respiratory tract inflammation
and licorice root, 89
and mint oil, 96
and peppermint, 112
and plantain, 114
and primrose, 118
and radish, 126
and sage, 134
and star anise seed, 145
and watercress, 157
See also Colds, flu, and bronchitis

Restlessness, and valerian root, 153. *See also* Anxiety, stress, and restlessness

Rheumatic problems
and eucalyptus, 45
and rosemary leaf, 132
and white willow bark, 159

Rheumatoid arthritis, and mistletoe, 98

Rhubarb root, 128–29

Rose flower, 130–31

Rose hips, 130, 180

Rosemary leaf, 132–33

Royal jelly, 63

Roybal, Beth Ann Petro
on damiana, 171
on fennel, 47
on sarsaparilla, 137
on yohimbe, 182

Saffron, 181

Sage, 134–35

St. John's wort, 141–44

Sarsaparilla, 136–37

Saw palmetto berry, 138–40

Scarlet fever, and belladonna, 7

Seasickness, and ginger, 56–57

Sexual problems
and fennel, 47
and sarsaparilla, 137

Side effects. *See specific herbs*

Skin irritations and problems
and flaxseed, 51
and sarsaparilla, 136
and witch hazel, 161

Skowronski, Gayle
on damiana, 171
on fennel, 47
on sarsaparilla, 137
on yohimbe, 182

Sleeping problems
and chamomile flower, 22
and hops, 71
and lavender, 85
and lemon balm, 87
and valerian root, 153, 154

Snake root (black cohosh root), 12–13

Spearmint oil, 96–97

Squaw root (black cohosh root), 12–13

Star anise seed, 145–46

Stomach cramps
and star anise seed, 145

Stomach problems
and anise seed, 5
and belladonna, 7–8
and bitter orange peel, 11
and caraway seed, 20
and chamomile flower, 22
and chicory, 24
and cinnamon bark, 26, 27
and dandelion, 34
and dill seed, 38
and fennel, 47
and flaxseed, 51
and ginger, 56
and haronga, 67
and juniper berry, 81
and lavender, 85
and licorice root, 89–90
and marshmallow, 91

and milk thistle fruit, 93
and peppermint, 112–13
and rosemary leaf, 132
and St. John's wort, 141
and star anise seed, 145
and turmeric root, 149
and yarrow, 163
Stress. *See* Anxiety, stress, and
restlessness
Succory (chicory), 24–25
Sunburn, and aloe, 3–4
Sweet balm (lemon balm), 87–88
Sweet mary (lemon balm), 87–88
Sweetweed (marshmallow), 91–92
Swendlow, Joel L.
on aloe, 3
on eucalyptus, 45
on valerian root, 153

Thomas, Samuel, 107
Throat problems
and anise seed, 5
and bilberry fruit, 9
and blackberry leaf, 14
and marshmallow, 91
and rose flower, 130
Thyme, 147–48
Thyroid problems
and belladonna, 7
and motherwort, 100
Time limits, for herb use, 188. *See
also specific herbs*
Tinnitus, and gingko biloba, 58
Toadpipe (horsetail herb), 79–80
Toothache, and cloves, 29
Turmeric root, 149–50
Tyler, Varro E.

on black cohosh root, 13
on borage, 170
on Commission E, xii
on devil's claw root, 36
on damiana, 171
on ephedra, 172–73
on hawthorn, 69
on juniper berry, 81
on mistletoe, 98
on parsley, 110
on peppermint, 112
on rosemary leaf, 132
on St. John's root, 141, 144
on valerian root, 153
on witch hazel, 161
on yohimbe, 182

Ulcers, contraindications, 186. *See
also* Stomach problems
Urinary problems
and cinnamon, 26
and goldenrod, 65
and horseradish, 77
and horsetail herb, 79
and parsley, 110
and pumpkin seed, 124
and saw palmetto berry, 138
and uva ursi leaf, 151
U.S., and herbal medicines, x
U.S. Food and Drug
Administration, x, xiii
Usage instructions. *See specific
herbs*
Uva ursi leaf, 151–52

Vaginal yeast infections, and echinacea, 40, 41

Valerian root, 153–56
Varicose veins
    and horse chestnut seed, 75
    and witch hazel, 161
Velvet plant (mullein flower),
    102–103
Vertigo, and ginkgo biloba, 58

Watercress, 157–58
Weights and measures chart,
    193
Weil, Andrew
    on aloe, 4
    on echinacea, 40, 43
    on valerian root, 154, 155
White willow bark, 159–60
Whooping cough, and thyme,
    147

Whortleberry (bilberry), 9–10
Wild thyme, 147
Winterbloom (witch hazel),
    161–62
Witch hazel leaf and bark,
    161–62
Wounds and wound healing
    and chamomile flower, 22
    and comfrey, 32
    and echinacea, 41
    and garlic, 53
    and horsetail herb, 79
    and witch hazel, 161
Woundwort (yarrow), 163–64

Yarrow, 163–64
Yeast (brewer's yeast), 16–17
Yohimbe, 182

ULYSSES PRESS MIND/BODY BOOKS

GIVE YOUR FACE A LIFT: NATURAL WAYS TO LOOK AND FEEL GOOD
Penny Stanway, $17.95
This full-color guide to natural face care tells how to give oneself a
"natural facelift" using oils, creams, masks and homemade products that
nourish and beautify the skin.

HEALING REIKI: REUNITE MIND, BODY AND SPIRIT
WITH HEALING ENERGY
Eleanor McKenzie, $16.95
Examines the meaning, attitudes and history of Reiki while providing
practical tips for receiving and giving this universal life energy.

HOW MEDITATION HEALS: A PRACTICAL GUIDE
TO IMPROVING YOUR HEALTH AND WELL-BEING
Eric Harrison, $12.95
Combines Eastern wisdom with medical and scientific evidence to ex-
plain how and why meditation improves the functioning of all systems
of the body.

HOW TO MEDITATE: AN ILLUSTRATED GUIDE
TO CALMING THE MIND AND RELAXING THE BODY
Paul Roland, $16.95
Offers a friendly, illustrated approach to calming the mind and raising
consciousness through various techniques, including basic meditation,
visualization, body scanning for tension, affirmations and mantras.

THE JOSEPH H. PILATES METHOD AT HOME: A BALANCE, SHAPE,
STRENGTH & FITNESS PROGRAM
Eleanor McKenzie, $16.95
This handbook describes and details Pilates, a mental and physical pro-
gram that combines elements of yoga and classical dance.

KNOW YOUR BODY: THE ATLAS OF ANATOMY
2nd edition, Introduction by Emmet B. Keeffe, M.D., $14.95
Provides a comprehensive, full-color guide to the human body.

NEW AGAIN!: THE 28-DAY DETOX PLAN FOR BODY AND SOUL
Anna Selby, $16.95
Allows you to free your body and mind from toxins and live a healthy
and balanced life.

SENSES WIDE OPEN: THE ART AND PRACTICE
OF LIVING IN YOUR BODY
Johanna Putnoi, $14.95
Through simple, accessible exercises, this book shows how to be at ease
with yourself and experience genuine pleasure in your physical connec-
tion to others and the world.

THE 7 HEALING CHAKRAS:
UNLOCKING YOUR BODY'S ENERGY CENTERS
Brenda Davies, $14.95
Explores the essence of chakras, vortices of energy that connect the
physical body with the spiritual.

SEX HERBS: NATURE'S SEXUAL ENHANCERS
Beth Ann Petro Roybal and Gayle Skowronski, $14.95
Presents detailed descriptions of safe, natural products that boost sexual
desire and pleasure.

SIMPLY RELAX: AN ILLUSTRATED GUIDE TO SLOWING DOWN
AND ENJOYING LIFE
Dr. Sarah Brewer, $15.95
In a beautifully illustrated format, this book clearly presents physical
and mental disciplines that show readers how to relax.

WEEKEND HOME SPA: FOUR CREATIVE ESCAPES—CLEANSING,
ENERGIZING, RELAXING AND PAMPERING
Linda Bird, $16.95
Not a book of face packs and detox diets nor a program of rigid
timetables, *Weekend Home Spa* offers practical treatments to cleanse,
energize, relax or shamelessly pamper. Holistic in approach, the book is
filled with everything from yoga exercises to funky dance moves,
health-minded recipes to expert tips on enhancing your well-being.

To order these books call 800-377-2542 or 510-601-8301, fax 510-
601-8307, e-mail ulysses@ulyssespress.com, or write to Ulysses Press,
P.O. Box 3440, Berkeley, CA 94703. All retail orders are shipped free
of charge. California residents must include sales tax. Allow two to
three weeks for delivery.

ABOUT THE AUTHOR

David Armstrong is a staff writer for the *San Francisco Chronicle*, where he covers the Pacific Rim region, international trade, and world travel, and writes a column on travel books for the travel section; he was formerly the editor of the *San Francisco Examiner*'s twice-weekly Health Page, which addressed health and medical issues. In addition, he has contributed articles to the *Village Voice*, *Los Angeles Times*, *Longevity*, *Travel & Leisure* magazine, *New York Times Syndicate*, *Toronto Globe & Mail*, and *Toronto Star*. Previously published books include *The Insider's Guide to Health Foods* (Bantam, 1984) and *The Great American Medicine Show* (Simon & Schuster, 1991), an illustrated history of alternative medicine in the United States. David lives in San Francisco, California.